FROM NOW ON

Easing and Transforming
Lives Interrupted by Illness or Injury

An Introduction to the Philosophy, Practices, and Processes of Sevenfold Healing and Cure

BETH ALDERMAN MD MPH

SEVENFOLD HEALING   SYSTEMS*MEDIA*GUILDS   SEATTLE

This book is an introductory text that describes a new paradigm for self-guided healing. It is not a substitute for the personal and immediately practical advice of a doctor, nor is the advice of a doctor a substitute for continuous self-care based on common sense and self-transformation. If you need help now, contact a suitable professional.

If your life has been interrupted by illness, injury, or other problems arising from the body, and you wish to begin practicing self-guided sevenfold healing, consult the second edition of the wisdom healing text entitled *The Chronic Illness Owner's Manual*, a workbook designed to support readers who are on the path to self-guided healing.

Sevenfold Healing Systems
An Imprint of Multifaith Witness Films and Books LLC
PO Box 45822
Seattle WA 98145-0822
http://7foldHealing.com; http://sevenfoldcure.com

ISBN #: 978-0-9820836-4-2

First Edition; First Printing, Sevenfold Healing Systems; Seattle.

To Ed, Eva, and Bryan

"Do what you can, where you are, with what you have."

~Theodore Roosevelt

Table of Contents

Preface

If your life has been interrupted by illness or injury, and you have passed through the crisis into a time of darkness, and you are ready to create a new life of healing and cure, this book is for you.

In this book, you will explore a new model of the body and new systems of healing and cure that I developed to guide my healing and cure from myalgic encephalomyelitis. This model and these systems grew out of my years of experience as a student of biology; a doctor of mainstream medicine; a specialist in public health and preventive medicine; an academic medical researcher; and a seeker of emotional and spiritual healing. You can use these systems in consultation with doctors, counselors, and bodyworkers who are supporting your healing and cure.

From Now On is transformational rather than inspirational, which means that it supports you to create dynamic changes in your body and your life. It features practices for healing and cure that seed processes of relief, wellbeing, transformation, and cure, defined in sevenfold healing as the creation of a new and better life.

When you were a toddler, you learned at an extraordinary pace by watching and mimicking your elders and by using trial and error to hone your senses, find your balance, and work with the world around you. As you grew up, formal education may have taught you to absorb vast amounts of information at the cost of turning you into a passive learner who relies heavily on classes, programs, and media.

When you practice sevenfold healing and cure, you can return to learning from experience as well as from others. As you do this, you can use the ideas and methods of sevenfold healing to observe your unfolding life, prudently alter it, observe the consequences, and gently alter it again. You can thus guide your healing and cure by learning from experience and from your doctors, counselors, and bodyworkers. When you guide yourself, you can heal inside and out and can embark on a new and better life.

The interruption in your life has given you the chance to form new patterns of living. You can take this chance to explore unforeseen breaks in habit or routine, unwanted limits or lacks in your sevenfold body, and the limits of human and natural systems. You can face the unknown and uncertain, address the tangible and intangible, and try new ways of thinking about your body and your life. As you do this, you may recognize that you are always creating a new life and that you can now create one that is better than any you have known in the past.

As you create your new life, you can take inspiration from the shared human history of transformation that you can find in ancient myths and fables; in the works of scientists like Newton, Da Vinci, Jenner, and Einstein; and in social change led by historic figures such as Addams, Muir, Hanh, Fukokua, and Maattai. You can discover ways to change and to change the ways that you change and thus advance your healing and cure.

As you consider sevenfold healing and cure, recognize that you are the healer and the curer of your life and that the offerings from Sevenfold Healing SYSTEMS*MEDIA*GUILDS are tools for you to use as you create healing and cure. If and when you encounter anything in these offerings that prompts harm, pass over it lightly and look for things that support your present processes of healing and cure. Trust yourself to know when and if to return to any passages that are wrong for you now.

May your healing be swift and easy
May your cure be dynamic and lasting
And may the sum of your experiences heal your sevenfold body and more

~Beth Alderman, 2013, Seattle

Part One:
Ideas and Methods

When your life is interrupted by illness or trauma, you may try to go on as you were. If this works well, you may devote little time or effort to your healing or cure; if it does not, you may seek help from a doctor. If you cannot access a doctor, or the doctor offers only limited help, you can use this book to help yourself.

In the pages that follow, you will meet a new idea of the body called the sevenfold paradigm, which supports self-guided systems of healing and cure. These systems include complete sets of practices for healing through relief, wellbeing, and transformation and for cure through the creation of a new life that is better than any you can presently imagine. These systems thus offer you the chance to create greater healing and cure than anyone could create for you.

As you practice sevenfold healing and cure, you learn to recognize, enter into, and abide in healing states of being and to strengthen healing habits and abilities that deepen, broaden, and extend your healing states. When your healing states have become strong and resilient, you can develop states, habits, and abilities of cure by which to create a new and better life one step at a time.

Because Sevenfold Healing Systems draw on ancient and modern traditions, they enable you to consult with doctors, counselors, and bodyworkers who hold widely divergent points of view. These systems also enable you to move beyond the limitations of modern systems so as to explore new frontiers of healing and cure.

In the first part of this book, you prepare for the practice of self-guided sevenfold healing and cure by becoming familiar with some of the key ideas and methods of sevenfold healing.

Chapter 1. The Sevenfold Model

Your sevenfold body is awesome. As long as you live, your body will sustain a multitude of exquisitely complex, miraculously joined, automatic processes that are dynamic and resilient, that is, that tend to remain in or to return to their usual state. Some of the processes are tangible while others are not; all tend to continue as they are, even in times of crisis. Because these processes join you to the web of life to which you belong, the resilience of your processes is joined with the vast reservoir of recovery and renewal that is arising from all sources of life.

To realize healing and cure in your body, you can actively shift your equilibrium from processes of death and destruction to those of life and creation. When you learn to do this, you can heal and cure your body from the inside out and so deepen your grounding in the web of life in time. To form a mental framework to hold the ideas of sevenfold healing, you can begin with the sevenfold model of the body.

A New Paradigm of the Body

When illness or trauma interrupts your life, your body responds in tangible and intangible ways that may be surprising and mysterious. Most of these responses fall outside the concrete objective thinking of modern science and the vague, subjective thinking of pre-modern philosophers. Even when you use all of the paradigms that support the work of your consultants, you may find that they do not enable you to create complete healing and cure.

The sevenfold model of the body offers a new way to view the body that simplifies what is complex in ways that are useful, complete, and practical. The sevenfold model is open and inclusive, so you can use it to bring in and unify other views of the body. In other words, it is an umbrella paradigm that supports self-guided healing and cure with complete sets of practices. The sevenfold model includes awareness, understanding, perceptions, sensations, energy, flesh, and interbeing, each of which is described below.

2

Flesh. The most familiar aspect of the sevenfold model of the body is the flesh, in which moderns found glimpses of the beautifully detailed intricacies of life that inspired and enabled scientists to develop many cures for disease. This very view of the flesh has also led scientists into mazes that go on forever or lead to dead ends. This view has also been used as the basis for many industries that are no longer sustainable. An old medical joke has it that the operation was a success but the patient died; a new one might be that the database included a perfect autopsy and a bill that will never be paid.

To make the most of what modern medical science can offer, you can consult a doctor who has committed a lifetime to studying and gaining experience in modern global medicine. When you have told your doctors about your intentions and expectations, you can join with them in finding your diagnosis, prognosis, and treatment and in learning from your progress and setbacks in healing and cure.

When you set out to guide the healing and cure of your flesh, you are like a small child with a chemistry set who likes the colors that appear when you fire a compound but who has no idea what the compound is or how the fire is produced; you need a mentor who can read the manual, supervise and share in your experiments, and help you to comprehend what you learn.

Interbeing. This least familiar aspect of the body is both tangible and intangible. It comprises your ties with the world around you, that is, with the web of life and the matrix of space and time. It is called interbeing after the thinking of Thich Nhat Hanh and reflects the dynamic continuity of all life explored through newer sciences such as ecology and population genetics.

If you think in scientific terms, you can see your interbeing in your interrelations with resources that circulate through the carbon and hydrologic cycles; with the sun's energy, which offers radiant heat and light to support photosynthesis; and with inorganic substrates such as minerals drawn from the earth's crust. You can also see your interbeing in your exchange of oxygen and carbon dioxide with plants; your intake and release of minerals that work with your enzymes; and your skin's use of sunlight to make active vitamin D. You can also see your interbeing as including your microbiome, that is, the two to five pounds of good germs that live in and with you and that you rely on to block infections, to make the nutrients you need, and to exchange with the good germs in the soil around you that nurture food crops and recycle night soil and compost.

If you think in spiritual terms, you can grasp interbeing through the poetic language of religious mystics who meditate on phenomena that range in scale from the infinitesimal to the infinite. Thich Nhat Hanh describes interbeing as an ocean and each being as a wave on the ocean. Mystics like Adam Frank and Brian Swimme, who are also theoretical physicists, are beginning to use spoken language to unite ideas derived indirectly by math and science with those discerned directly through meditation and contemplation.

Your part of interbeing also joins your body with space and time. Thus, to guide the healing and cure of your sevenfold body you can see it as made up of sets of overlapping, ephemeral processes that are always in motion and that have effects that add up over your lifetime. Rather than seeing your healing and cure as episodic, you can see them as ongoing processes through which you create healing and cure in sync with life in space and time.

Through your part of interbeing, you have a particular place in the history of life on earth, which includes states and habits of harm and healing that come into you from outside and that may be as important as those that arise in you with experience. You thus hold what sevenfold healing conceives of as time debts, that is, processes of harm that you can pay or forgive to ease your healing and cure.

For example, your family or community may have suffered trauma that became a part of the past that lives on in your sevenfold body as harmful states and habits and that you can transform through healing. Likewise, the web of life around you may be suffering damage that lives in you as tangible and intangible damage to your interbeing, including your microbiome, and that you can help to resolve by joining with others to restore your habitat or a remnant of the wilds that serve as storehouses of healing and cure.

The legacy that you leave behind after this life arises from your part of interbeing. That is, the sum total of your processes of healing and cure plus your processes of harm equals your imprint on life in time. If you leave before your time, or do not pay or forgive your time debts, or do not become a source of healing and cure, your legacy will likely be a burden to the web of life. To complete your life and to leave the best of yourself as your legacy, you can become a source of healing and cure and leave the world a better place.

When you heal and cure your interbeing, you are like a wise elder who cares well for self and others for a many good years before putting in order the affairs of a lifetime, providing for the support and care of the young, blessing each and every source of life, and putting aside worldly cares to rest in joy before resting in peace.

Sensations. The most tangible connection between your flesh and its surroundings is the aspect of the body known in sevenfold healing as sensations, which includes the five senses of sight, hearing, taste, smell, and touch; the inner ear's sense of acceleration and position; the pineal gland's ability to detect light and darkness; the senses of pain, cold, heat, and pressure in the skin and position in the joints; as well as ineffable senses mediated by energy, as when you sense someone staring at you. Sensations also include sense awarenesses, that is, senses that you construct, hone, and interpret such as perfect pitch, a cultivated palate, or recognition of optical illusions.

Because sensations can distract you, your elders may have taught you to be wary of pleasant sensations or to rely on austerity to stay on task and on track. When your life is interrupted, such negative views of sensations can undermine your healing and cure. To engage their healing possibilities, you can shift your attention away from sensations that prompt harmful states and habits and toward those that prompt states and habits of healing and cure.

For example, pleasing sensations may prompt relief or wellbeing, as when you take a hot bath to relax tense muscles or ease stiff joints or when you use a pleasing fragrance, soft pillow, or healing touch to offset discomfort. You can also learn to read your sensations so as to avoid harmful states and habits, as when you cover your ears

5

to block out airplane noise and temper any increase in blood pressure, or you note that a hard pillow is giving you a headache and switch to a soft one. As you advance in sevenfold healing, you can use sensations to monitor your body and, with practice, to align your healing and cure with your present circumstances.

Sensations link your flesh to near and distant surroundings, as when a loud street noise prompts tension, a foul smell triggers a gag reflex, the dark days of winter induce sleep, or a change in the weather hurts your joints. You can use this connection between your body and your surroundings to find sources of relief and wellbeing and to monitor your healing and cure.

When you work well with sensations, you are like a an air traffic controller who can take in signals, pay attention to the right ones at the right time, make good choices, and respond so as to allow airplanes to come and go without doing them harm.

Energy. Energy is useful in healing and cure because your energy body can bypass new limits of the flesh and can catalyze healing transformation. In sevenfold healing, you can think of energy as including the electrical and magnetic activity of your flesh and as the subtle, dynamic, and resilient skeleton of the intangible body. The energy body has a subtle structure that parallels the brain and spinal cord as well as the nerves, ganglia, and nexi of the autonomic nervous system, which serves your digestive system and other organ systems.

Modern medicine has yet to engage the energy body in healing or cure. While modern medical science has developed tests such as the electrocardiogram, electroencephalogram, and electromyelogram, and procedures such as cardiac ablation and cochlear implants, it offers few useful means for using the energy body in self-guided healing and cure. This may be for the best; no device can be as finely attuned to your state of being or guide its response as well as your sevenfold body.

When you work with your energy body, you become familiar with your central channel, which runs along the front of your spine, and the energy centers, the most important of which lie in that channel at the levels of the crown, throat, heart, solar plexus, navel, and sacrum. In Sanskrit, the central channel is called the shushumna nadi and the centers are called chakras, that is, wheels.

When you learn to heal and cure your energy body, and through your energy body to catalyze the healing and cure of the rest of your sevenfold body, you are like an artist of the future who is designing an intangible kinetic sculpture that is beautiful, dynamic, and translucent and has a flexible, strong axis with wheels that spin constantly to circulate energy through areas of need. You design this sculpture with your mind, place it inside your flesh at the front of your spine, and support it to mediate your healing intentions and to discern and transform your states and habits of harm.

Perceptions. This aspect of the sevenfold body acts as a gateway between the above-listed levels and your understanding. Its purpose is to devote your understanding to what is most important by excluding useless data and responding automatically to familiar situations. These automatic responses range from conditioned reflexes, such as taking your hand from a hot stove, to primary reactive postures, such as roles of pleasing or pushing, to the store of complex habitual responses that you began to form in early childhood and continue to use today. Your gateway thus frees your understanding to focus on the three to seven factors that interest you in the moment.

Chances are good that this gateway has become so familiar to you that you take it as your identity and rely on it to make most of your decisions. Now, when your life has been interrupted by illness or injury, you will want to open your filter to admit new clues to healing and cure and to respond to present conditions rather than to the conditions of your childhood.

Chances are also good that the interruption in your life has revealed flaws in your old gateway. You may discover that your automatic perceptions prompt more harmful states and habits than healing ones. You may note patterns of response to self, others, and the web of life that feature harmful states of fear, hatred, greed, apathy, or dissociation and that those states go with habits that undermine healing and cure. You may note that your sevenfold healing and cure will depend on the healing of your perceptions.

To heal your perceptions, you can begin to favor responses that prompt healing states and habits and pay less attention to those that prompt harmful states and habits. As you advance, and become able to transform harmful responses into healing ones, you can create a new, open, dynamic gateway that admits whatever may be of most use in the moment. You can use this new gateway to support your healing and cure with states of contentment, delight, and happiness.

You may find it more difficult to heal perceptions than to heal or cure any other aspect of your body. One reason for this is your perceptions are, by nature, hidden from your awareness. They are also fast and joined with other aspects of the body, including the energy body that tends to sustain them. To heal perceptions, you can work gently and creatively and play with many methods until you find those that are right for you.

One type of method that can be effective is group work. Group work requires prudence because it can be subject to error and abuse. It requires clear personal intentions, strong healing states, and specific skills. One skill is being able to discern and sustain the right degree of openness and effort in the moment as too little will yield nothing while too much may do harm.

As you heal your perceptions, and learn to use your perceptions to further healing and cure, your old patterns may be tenacious and your new ones elusive. To get help with these difficulties, you can consult a counselor who is experienced, ethical, and suited to you as you are now. Whether you work on your own or with a counselor, you can become able to create and abide in strong healing states and to create healing habits and abilities as described in *Part Two*.

When you heal and cure your perceptions, you are like a corporate manager who is responsible for creating procedures for workers to follow and who is always observing the accuracies and errors that arise from the procedures and from the workers' use of them. That is, when things are working well, you leave them as they are; when you note misuse of time, effort, or other resources, you can revise your procedures and retrain your workers, consulting with others as desired. Then, when circumstances change, you can adapt so as to continue allocating resources wisely.

Understanding. Your understanding enables you to see new patterns and to grasp new paradigms and possibilities—that is, to apprehend and comprehend new things. With a strong understanding, you can take meaning from life and use meaning to guide your healing and cure. You can recognize the familiar, use words and numbers, develop trains of thought, and devise sensible courses of action.

If you had formal schooling, you may have habits of understanding that you can use for healing and cure. You may have habits of following, absorbing, and repeating trains of thought by which to form new insights and perspectives, to devise strategies and plans, and to join with your consultants and systems of care in effecting your goals as you take charge of your sevenfold body.

If you had formal schooling, you may also have developed some habits that you may wish to unlearn. For example, you may have learned to absorb the written word instead of making sense of your experience. Or you may have disciplined your understanding at the expense of the rest of your sevenfold body, as when you sit still too long, take in too much data, repeat trains of thought too often, or hold fixed ideas. You may have learned to mistrust your experience or become unable to hone your common sense.

If you did not have formal schooling, or your understanding is weak, you can strengthen it in the way of self-taught scholars like Abraham Lincoln. That is, you can read and discuss texts that support healing and cure and find mentors who can show you how to use those texts to guide yourself. You can use what you learn to note and appreciate inborn healing abilities and to form and guide dynamic processes of cure. You can learn to find, to try out, and to size up new ways of healing and cure. You can develop habits by which to use your experience to hone your common sense.

9

Your understanding is like your perceptions in that it will be weak if it is concrete and fixed and thus prone to reflecting the past rather than the present and thereby prone to going out of sync with life in time. It will also be weak if it is too flimsy or too unstructured and thus likely to fall apart in times of need. Your understanding lies beyond the gateway of perceptions and so is more open to awareness and easier to bring up to speed. It is made up of worldviews, ideas, and rules that you can see and change to support your healing and cure.

When you heal your understanding you are like a teen who lives at the beach and who envisions and builds sand castles that give form to the shifting sands. Whenever the tide sweeps a castle away, the teen envisions and builds another that the elements soon reclaim, allowing the teen a chance to re-envision and re-build anew.

Consciousness. The least tangible aspect of your sevenfold body is consciousness, that is, awareness. You can focus your awareness as attention and concentration and so create a foreground that is like a magnifying lens that can penetrate and influence any aspect of the sevenfold body. While the background of your healthy awareness is even, unobstructed, and boundless, your focus can zoom in on the tiniest particle, take in the face of a beloved friend, or encompass a galaxy of stars that brightens the night sky.

Consciousness is like the space that you embody and therefore includes all levels of the sevenfold body. With healing and cure, this space becomes free of irregularities, discontinuities, or boundaries and supports your understanding in the healing of your perceptions and all other levels of the sevenfold body. By remaining strongly centered and rooted in this space, you can avoid wasting resources on boundaries that children may form for concealment or for self-protection and that may later constrict healing or cure.

When you heal awareness, the space you embody extends outward and attenuates without being limited in space or time. You heal awareness when your body is alert, relaxed, and grounded and when you can recognize, enter into, and sustain healing states in which to practice processes that deepen, broaden, and extend your states and habits of healing and cure. As your awareness heals, it becomes able to support your understanding to detect and transform obstacles to healing and cure and to take steps toward cure that bring you into closer sync with life in time as you create a new and better life that fulfills your ultimate purpose.

When you heal your consciousness, you are like a food truck owner whose truck is damaged by a flood, and who clears out and cleans up the truck so as to continue sharing recipes new and old.

New Definitions of Healing and Cure

While attempting to heal from myalgic encephalomyelitis, I came to define healing as the ongoing realization of relief, wellbeing, and transformation. To support this realization, I developed Sevenfold Healing Systems and designed them to support self-guided healers in learning to recognize, enter into, and abide in healing states of being and to develop healing habits and abilities to strengthen those states. If you practice self-guided healing, you can use Sevenfold Healing Systems to be and to become healing, that is, to rest in healing states in the moment and to deepen, broaden, and extend those states over time.

When my healing states had become strong enough to support cure, I came to define cure as the creation of a new and dynamic life that fulfills your ultimate purpose and is always becoming better than any you previously imagined. To create this life, you abide in healing states as you develop states, habits, and abilities of cure to use in finding components of cure and bringing them into your new life. While you may assess inward healing and cure directly and subjectively, you also assess outward healing and cure indirectly and objectively, that is, from the perspective of life in time.

This definition of cure is unlike that of the late modern era, when cure was seen as the end of fleshly evidence of disease. This definition was rooted in Vesalius' objective study of anatomy and shaped by Napoleon's adoption of technologies such as Jenner's vaccine to protect "valid" lives, that is, the lives of soldiers. Viewing medicine in the context of the military paradigm led doctors to use force against agents of disease and to expect collateral damage, rescue, and reconstruction. These expectations shaped the complex systems of late modern medical care, which managers engineered to deliver usual, customary, and reasonable practices and to impose quality controls and accounting procedures. These led to excessive uniformity and conformity, fixed care as it was, and leveled care by bring up substandard care and bringing down superior care.

If your perceptions of healing and cure conform to popular ideas of crisis and response, you may expect medical care to offer scenarios of thrilling resuscitations, cancer cures that snatch patients from the jaws of death, and high-tech repairs of anatomical injuries. If you also accept the consumer model of temporary relief and lasting dependence, you may find it very difficult to believe that you can create your own healing and cure.

On the other hand, you may take easily to self-guided sevenfold healing and cure if you think of healing and cure as restoring your inner habitat; or as a spiritual journey or quest; or as the step-by-step, iterative, and inventive assembly of raw materials into a prototype vehicle that you can drive to freedom. You may be ready to resume your authority and responsibility for your sevenfold body and for your healing and cure if you know others whose lives were interrupted and who used their ingenuity, common sense, faith, and experience to create new and better lives.

New Approaches to Healing and Cure

If you have participated in a system of modern global medical care, you will have surrendered much of your responsibility and authority to that system. When that system comes to your aid and cures you swiftly and effectively without harming you, you may rest content. When it does not, you may wish to take charge of your sevenfold body. You may see that you can learn to know your body directly as no one else can and that you are thus best qualified to guide your own healing and cure.

If you choose to use a Sevenfold Healing System in consultation with your doctors, counselors, and bodyworkers, you can follow steps like those outlined in *Part Two* below and presented in detail in the upcoming second edition of *The Chronic Illness Owner's Manual*. Because Sevenfold Healing Systems are new, they may be best for those with the pioneering spirit to engage their horse sense, time, effort, and ingenuity in relieving and transforming the wondrous, mutable body as they help to develop the resources noted below.

Systems. Each Sevenfold Healing System includes a complete set of sequential, synergistic practices that seed processes of healing and cure and engage your creativity and dynamism. As you learn a practice through the exercises, you learn how to create relief and wellbeing by recognizing, entering into, and abiding in healing states of being; by forming healing habits that awaken and develop your inborn healing abilities; by resolving your time debts by paying or forgiving them; and by healing with your habitat. You also learn to transform harmful states and habits as you transform your life.

The exercises of sevenfold healing rely on age-old and new esoteric practices that grew out of pre-modern as well as modern ideas of the body. These practices use meditative skills such as visualization; practices in daily life such as working questions; and habits of cure that support ongoing empirical learning. Most predate or postdate the modern struggle between religious and scientific authorities that puts the tangible and objective against the intangible and subjective.

As may be obvious, doing the inner work of healing and cure does not follow the present model of procuring instant relief by buying a pill or obtaining a device or a procedure. Inner work relies on active, dynamic intentions; strong, flexible motivations; daily practice; and pre-modern virtues such as patience and persistence. In sevenfold healing, you can do this work as you partner with consultants who prescribe modern treatments. In other words, Sevenfold Healing Systems include intangible processes of healing and cure as well as tangible treatments of the flesh and interbeing.

At first, your intangible healing may be undetectable or subtle and evident only to you. As you progress, others who are sensitive or empathetic will begin to respond differently to you. Over time, you may show tangible results that doctors and scientists may be able to measure. When you become a source of healing and cure, you can share your healing and cure with others and with interbeing.

Your self-guided healing and cure will be like ascending a spiral staircase on which you sometimes pause or retrace your steps. With time, you can follow this staircase as far as Sevenfold Healing Systems will take you and then choose to enjoy your life as it is or to continue your ascent by repeating your work with a Sevenfold Healing System or by devising a system of your own.

Media. The system for chronic illness is detailed in the upcoming second edition of *The Chronic Illness Owner's Manual* (*Manual*) and in the *Healing Studio*, which will include *From Now On*, the *Manual*, and audio guides to the exercises. Systems for infertility, time debts, and habitat restoration are in development.

The *Manual* includes anecdotes, comments, exercises, and discussion questions that seed processes the reader can use to be and to become healing and cure. It also includes inspirational quotes and references to other resources. The *Manual* is in the form of a wisdom text; that is, it opens you to the unknown and unseen, catalyzes your self-transformation, and prepares you to create a new and better life.

Sevenfold Healing Media approach your illness, healing, and cure as unique in that they reflect the sum total of the life experience that is imprinted in your body. The Media support you to transform those experiences that live on in you as harmful states or habits, to leave behind those that are useless or distracting, and to strengthen those that support your healing states, habits, and abilities. The Media also prepare you to continuously monitor and change your sevenfold body so as to remain in sync with life in time and to be and become healing and cure for the sake of self and others.

Sevenfold Healing Media are for transformation rather than for inspiration. That is, they model the change from harmful states and habits to healing ones. In that way, the Media are interactive; that is, they assume your active and wise participation. For example, when the *Manual* addresses tough topics, you may respond with harmful states or habits that you are not yet ready to transform for use in healing and cure. Because no two people will respond alike, it will be up to you to note and skip over material that you are not ready to work with and to return to it if and when you deem it right.

Likewise, if you know that you tend to take on too little or too much, you can take particular care to exert right effort, that is, a degree of effort that falls between slacking and striving. If you tend to shift your body's pain and suffering onto others, you can take care to relieve and to transform it yourself; if you tend to take on the pain and suffering of others, you can focus on that which is arising from your body. If you experience pain of the flesh, you can take care not to respond to it in a way that worsens it.

Sevenfold Healing Media are designed for individuals in search of healing and cure. If you are a doctor, counselor, or bodyworker, or you have an interest in supporting self-guided sevenfold healing and cure, you can do the exercises so as to transform your life and thereby gain the direct experience needed to grasp Sevenfold Healing Systems. Sevenfold Healing Media are designed to free self-guided healers and their consultants of the constraints that limit systems of care, such as the habits and expectations of third parties.

When you use a manual from Sevenfold Healing Media, you are like a composer who creates a theme for each process of healing and cure, who then sequences and combines those themes so as to discern dissonance and resolve it into harmony, and who then, in the reverb that follows the finish, can hear the music of the spheres.

Consultation. As part of being and becoming healing and cure, you learn to work with and so to access the expertise offered by your consultants and by your complex systems of care. Consultants who have committed their lives to the study and practice of a chosen discipline can help you to access the shared wisdom of the past as well as the latest results of research and development. When you engage a Sevenfold Healing System, you may have reason to consult doctors, counselors, and bodyworkers, as described in *Part Two, Chapters 2* and *4*.

15

The long-range vision of Sevenfold Healing includes the formation of Guilds. The Founders' Guild will be open to licensed allopathic doctors who are leaders in their chosen fields and who will help to develop the Masters' Guild. The Masters' Guild will be open to licensed allopathic doctors who take full training in Sevenfold Healing and Cure and who earn and maintain their certification as Masters. The Guides' Guild will be open to doctors, counselors, bodyworkers, and self-guided healers who take some training in Sevenfold Healing and Cure and who earn and maintain their certification as Guides. For now, you can best support your self-guided healing and cure by consulting doctors, counselors, and bodyworkers whom you like and who are willing to support you.

Chapter 2. The Upward Spiral

Now that you have sketched the framework of sevenfold healing and cure in your mind, you are ready to sketch in some of its basic steps. You can begin by orienting the first phase of your sevenfold healing and cure to the present time in history and by previewing the first steps of sevenfold healing and cure. As you do this, you are like a visitor to a museum who steps back to look at a timeline of history and then steps forward to focus on the now and to ponder the paradigms and possibilities that lie ahead of you.

Transition and Opportunity

Your life has been interrupted at a time when society is changing; the good news is that you can change with it. Society follows cycles, as when the age of discovery sparked the modern era and the age of romance began the late modern era. Now, at the end of the late modern era, you can gain perspective on the present moment by looking back on selected milestones in medical history. These milestones can mark the way to new frontiers of healing and cure that you can explore and to new opportunities that you can try.

In ancient times, doctors around the world saw the body as made up of basic elements such as air, fire, earth, and water. More than two millennia ago, Hippocrates and his followers transformed the ancient lineage of allopathy with the theory that the body was made up of four humors—blood, phlegm, yellow bile, and black bile. This theory enabled them to study the body objectively and to treat the body more systematically. They developed new modes of practice that they supported with the code of ethics that we know today as the Hippocratic Oath.

Ancient allopaths faced deadly diseases such as those we glimpse in the pages of Ovid's *Metamorphoses*, in which he notes a devastating plague at Aegina and a plague in Rome that prompted city leaders to appeal to a serpent god from Greece. Fortunately, we can see allopathy move beyond its limits again and again, as in the Late Middle Ages when Maimonides reconciled Abrahamic and Greek writings, and in the Renaissance when Vesalius broke the taboo against dissecting cadavers and gained accurate knowledge of anatomy.

Modern Lights. When doctors applied the modern tools of science to human ailments, they began to break through barriers to healing and cure at a fast pace. Jenner, Snow, Shattuck, Fleming, and others developed vaccines and hygiene programs that curbed the plagues that evolved with our species. Their modern methods became so effective that the practice of allopathy spread around the globe and enabled doctors in all countries to save and prolong countless lives and to cure our species of one ancient scourge, namely, smallpox.

Modern Shadows. The modern paradigm that enabled great gains is now limiting progress. One limitation is our inability to view healing and cure on a human scale. After the invention of devices like the microscope and telescope, we lost our sense of focus in labyrinths of baffling detail and in the vastness of space and time. Excessive attention to molecular biology has further diverted our focus from the body and the web of life. To restore your common sense, you can use the sevenfold paradigm to view the body on a human scale and follow fields such as zoology, botany, and ecology to enhance your understanding of the web of life in time.

Another limit to progress is the modern zeal for social engineering, through which we used fixed ideas and methods to form complex systems of care that ignore the intangible or difficult to measure;

that treat dynamic living systems as fixed, artificial ones; that distort healing and cure by tying them to money and power; and that focus on the virtual patient, that is, on the medical database rather than on life itself. This zeal has pushed cure into the background, multiplied costs, obstructed progress, and divided doctors from real life.

To pass through these barriers, you can focus on what matters even when it is intangible or difficult to measure. You can center your recovery in your body, focus on long-term results, and devote your time and effort to complete and lasting healing and cure.

Another limitation created by modernity is the fragmentation that results when analysis is not followed by synthesis. For example, Descartes divided human understanding from the rest of the body by defining life as thought. Later, Freud, Jung, and James divided the intangible aspects of the body from the tangible ones, and shunted care of the intangible into fields such as psychology and psychiatry. You can offset modern fragmentation by using the sevenfold paradigm to simplify complexity in a new way and try new and dynamic processes of analysis and synthesis.

Another barrier created by modernity is the tendency to make top-down systems that get too big—that is, to create complex systems and to centralize them. As these modern systems draw more and more care into medical centers, they divide doctors from patients' lives and from the web of life. They also foster the proliferation of subspecialties; the fixing and narrowing of algorithms of care; and the exclusion of the poor and of problems that modernity addresses poorly or not at all.

Modern systems also burdened practices of healing and cure with expectations of stable, long-term profits that require stasis and predictability and that form strong incentives to sustain illness and disability. In other words, late modern economies depend more and more on continued suffering and lifelong dependence on drugs and devices. Modern media foster this suffering and dependence by spreading harmful habits of response such as fear and greed and by drawing attention to products that offer ephemeral relief and divert attention from the slow and sure means of healing and cure that are freely available to all.

To pass through this barrier, you can join with others to support grass roots healing, select forms of healing and cure that yield true lasting benefit, and avoid memes that prompt harm. You can take a big picture view of your place in time.

You can penetrate all of these barriers by using the sevenfold paradigm and sevenfold systems of healing and cure to transform your life; to sync with life in time; to consult doctors who work well with you and with your counselors and bodyworkers; and to ground your healing and cure in interbeing as described in *Part Two*.

Emerging Possibilities. Because the limits of modern global medicine are becoming evident everywhere, and because healers around the globe are exploring new forms of healing and cure, you may be able to consult people who can share skills in indigenous, Eastern, or new medical traditions such as shamanism, acupuncture, yoga, Qi Gong, chiropractic, and homeopathy. When you do, you may receive conflicting advice. You may find that your carers are like the blind men and the elephant; that is, each sees only one aspect of the body and denies all others. You may find that it is up to you to make sense of the whole. To find out if this system may be right for you now, you can look over the steps below and try the exercises in *Part Two*.

Acceptance of Interruption

When you life has been interrupted, you may try to resume your usual patterns of being and becoming, that is, your usual state of being and your habits of changing that state. When this strategy is not useful, you face the challenge of accepting that your old habits no longer serve your needs and that they may even be interfering with your healing and cure. Acceptance enables you to look at new possibilities, to try new ways of living, and to form a new life that fulfills your purpose and that is better than the old one.

When you accept and embrace the present just as it is, you are like a long-distance runner who finds in mid-race that the old training program is not working and who stops for respite and refreshment before starting in on a new one.

Preparation for Self-Guidance

If you are used to freedom, authority, and responsibility, self-guided healing and cure may come as second nature to you; if you are used to taking a narrower role in a group or institution, it may seem odd or daunting. Either way, when you guide yourself or, rather, see that you are always guiding yourself, you will become able to take stock of your sevenfold body and your life and to take charge of your relief, wellbeing, transformation, and cure.

When you knowingly take hold of your life, you become aware that you can refuse care that will not help you and that you can join with your consultants and your systems of care in finding any care that will help you. You can do this better when you take a big picture view of your situation, stay open to new insights and perspectives, actively discern your problems, and engage in a prudent process of trial and error that leads you all the way to healing and cure.

For example, you may find that the web of life is not as you expect it to be, as when your food is harming you. Rather than consult doctors who may know little about the web of life, you can cut your diet back to foods you can count on, then add foods back one by one, and continue eating those that do not harm you. You do not need to rely on any entity to do this; you can create your healing or cure on your own or with others who share your difficulties.

Similarly, you may come to see that your past is contributing to your present pain and suffering, as when you note that troubling memories and unresolved problems prompt harmful state or habits. You can come to know your body and your life so well that you can put the past to rest and use the energy you thereby free to be and become healing and to form a legacy of healing and cure.

You can also slow down your automatic habits and change any that are working against your healing or cure. As you do this, you can disengage from habits that keep things running smoothly but that are useless or bad for you. You can then form dynamic new habits that are good for you and also keep things running smoothly as you realize healing and cure and adapt to changing circumstances.

When you guide your healing and cure, you observe your life, learn from it, and bring to bear all that you know and all that you learn to heal and cure your sevenfold body and your life. As you do this, you hone healing states, habits, and abilities like kindness, ingenuity, and creativity that improve your life in ways that may be subtle and gradual but that will make all the difference.

Dynamic Intentions and Expectations

When your life is interrupted by illness or trauma, chances are good that you will go through a series of changes, some of which may be abrupt and unsettling and some of which will be gradual and at times disheartening. If you have begun in crisis, and have used your resources and abilities to stabilize your life, you have created the chance to create new intentions and expectations that are dynamic, strong, and resilient and that will lead you through any and all of the welcome and unwelcome experiences that lie ahead on your way to sevenfold healing and cure.

When you use a Sevenfold Healing System, your intentions will be to realize relief, wellbeing, and transformation as you create a new and better life that fulfills your deepest purpose. You can then tailor your expectations to reflect your changing circumstances, that is, to form and to sustain realistic expectations that change with your healing and cure. These dynamic expectations will enable you to adapt your priorities as you learn to abide in deeper healing states and to shift your baseline state toward healing and cure.

If you have already honed your common sense, you may find it easy to form dynamic intentions and expectations. If not, you can use this interruption in your life to hone it so that you can tell what is urgent and what is important and balance them as needed. For example, if you lose your income, you may face urgent material needs that will take up all of your time and energy. When you have met those needs, you can return to the equally important task of finding your healing and creating your cure.

When you have formed strong, dynamic, and resilient intentions and expectations, no obstacle can deter you from healing or cure. You will be like a mountain climber who is using a rope, harness, and anchors to ascend a mountain by a chosen route and who is using abilities like ingenuity, balance, and strength to turn the folds and wrinkles of the rock's surface into handholds and footholds that lead to a place where nothing will be hidden and your purpose will be fulfilled.

Formation of Habits of Healing and Cure

When you are free to devote your time and attention to healing and cure, you will be ready to create a formal daily healing practice in which you strengthen and enhance your healing states, habits, and abilities; to put harmful states and habits to rest; to resolve your debts to life in time; and to create your new dynamic and fulfilling life. If illness or injury weakened one or more of the abilities on which you have relied in the past, you can use your daily healing practice to strengthen and enhance your habits of healing and cure, beginning with right effort, altruism, compassion, and integration.

As you develop your healing abilities with exercises like those in *Part Two* below and in the second edition of the *Manual*, you will learn to be healing, that is, to abide in healing states; and to become healing, that is, to deepen, broaden, extend, and share those states. You will also develop habits of cure that you can use to change your life. Your new ways of being, becoming, and living will then enable you to do the hard work of transforming your harmful states and habits as well as the delicate work of leaving behind those that are useless or wasteful.

As your abilities grow and develop, you will find out which you can use for what, and when and how you can use them. You learn to call on abilities that seed and support your processes of healing and cure, including abilities that you have neglected in the past and that will be just what you need to find new possibilities for healing and to create fresh ways of living. You will become healing, that is, you will embody the art of healing and cure.

22

As you form new habits of healing and cure, you are like a gardener who goes to a place where an old garden dried out and who clears away debris, brings in a source of water, renews the soil with worms and compost, and, when everything is ready, designs garden beds that suit the present moment and lays in and nurses the new garden. Later, as times change, the gardener renews the garden again and again so that it is always right for the here and now.

Transformation and Retirement of Habits of Harm

When your sevenfold body is burdened with harmful states and habits, you can transform them and so seed and support your healing and cure. When you have transformed one such habit, you can transform others and, in time, transform your whole life. With each transformation, you free up bodily resources that become available to your processes of healing and cure. Put differently, you can take any and all of your harmful states and habits as chances to be and to become healing and cure.

When you have identified a state or habit that burdens your body, such as an intense state of anger, fear, or craving, you can take it as a signal that there is something that you should be doing that you haven't yet done. Some part of your sevenfold body is aware and is signaling you as best it can. Chances are that you have ignored a concern for a very long time and that ignoring it is tying up your resources and limiting your healing and cure. Once you know what it is, you will be able to bring to bear on it all the abilities of your sevenfold body and all the threads of your life. If you have many such habits, you may feel for a while like a Mad Hatter with a list that can't wait.

For example, you can look deeply into the habit and detect hidden sources of distress that are keeping it alive. As you study it closely, you form new insights and perspectives that show you the source of the distress and ways to ease it. That is, rather than sustain a state that is like taking poison and waiting for someone else to die, you can pinpoint the sources of the state, address them directly, and release their energy for healing and cure. As the poet Rilke put it, you can see your dragons as princesses waiting to be kissed, that is,

23

as valued parts of yourself that you have hidden away as if in a tower and that are longing for you to brave the barriers so that you can embrace them and release them from bondage.

You can begin seeding processes of transformation by forming simple, new, tangible habits, as when you use a walking stick or cane to steady new imbalance, or use a talking book after losing your vision, or keep to a cast after breaking your leg. When you have seeded processes of change, you can begin to change less tangible habits of harm such as guilt, shame, or blame. If any habit sticks, as may be the case if it was set through early or repeated upset, you can use the exercises in *Part Two* or in the *Manual* or you can enlist the aid of a consultant or mentor. With prudence and right effort, you can become able to transform any habit, however harmful.

When you change your habits, you are like a person who has built a house of cards and is taking them back so as to build another. You keep cards that symbolize habits that you value and exchange others for new ones you are trying out. As you create your healing and cure, you build and rebuild your house until it includes only those cards that are holding their value and that you expect may do so as time passes.

Part Two:
Sevenfold Practices and Processes

To be and to become healing, you undertake a formal daily practice in which to seed and nurture processes of healing and cure. If you follow a Sevenfold Healing System, you seed a complete set of processes that become second nature and that bring you into sync with life in time. As things change, or new habits of harm arise, you can use those practices or devise new ones to seed and to sustain needed processes of healing and cure.

When you practice your healing and cure, you are like a building manager who keeps a close eye on the structure and tenants of the building: the manager can recruit good tenants, call for services and repairs, network with neighbors, spot and evict problem tenants, and create a pleasant and welcoming atmosphere that puts everyone at ease and, while doing all of this, the manager is always learning and always improving.

Chapter 1. Healing States

Learning to abide in healing states is like learning to sing a song. You begin by listening to it and imagining the pitch and harmony you will create when you sing it. You then try it, listen to the results, and try again until you create and enjoy the pitch and harmony you imagined. If you are gifted or skilled, you may do this quickly. If not, you can practice and so nurture your abilities as you develop specific skills.

You begin to work with healing states by learning to recognize them. You can do this by noticing the feelings of relief and wellbeing that you enjoy as they arise, as may happen in times of comfort or ease. You can also use a form of dynamic meditation or bodywork such as yoga, healing touch, Qi Gong, Reiki, or massage to invite you sevenfold body to enter into healing states that you can then study as you enjoy them. If you can access a bodyworker, you can also ask for direct, personal aid in learning to recognize, enter into, and abide in healing states that you can later create on your own and, as you gain skill, enhance as you wish.

If you find it difficult to identify healing states of being, you can take note of times when you feel good, as when you sense that you have come home or when you feel comfort, contentment, shelter, ease, or happiness. In a light healing state you may feel as if you are on retreat from the day's cares, or reliving a treasured moment, or refreshing your body and your life in a place of retreat. In a deep healing state you may feel as if the earth is opening its abundant wonders to your sevenfold body; as if a trusted elder or dear friend is thinking of you, loving you, and caring for you; or a divine being is taking joy in your ephemeral but unique and precious existence.

Learning to recognize healing states is like finding meaning in art; that is, your understanding can take you to a point where you can break through understanding, as with paradox or surprise. Learning to recognize healing states is also like feeling sound or writing with your other hand. You can feel it in the body as something that is already there and yet cannot be imposed by rote or reason.

If you have ignored healing states for a long time, they may have become elusive, uneven, or weak. It may take some time to discern the changeable, ineffable states that will support and enhance your processes of healing and cure. To ease your way, you can develop readiness, grounding, relaxation, focus, resilience, and strength on each level of the sevenfold body.

Readiness

At the level of awareness, readiness allows you to move the focus of your attention and concentration to any point in space and time and to rest it there. Ready awareness is thus free of densities or blanks as well as of blocks and boundaries. You can compare it to an unclouded sky, a deep and clear pool, or the nothingness from which all wonders arises. You can describe it as transparent, unimpeded, infinite, seamless, whole, or wide open.

You can expect your ready awareness to develop at the right time and at the right speed to support your unique course of healing and cure. If you like, you can approach it as you might immersion in the ocean, that is, as standing on the shore, trying the water with your toes, and slowly walking into the water until you are free to float and swim and explore and play like a seal who has come home.

A ready understanding is open to possibilities that lie beyond the modern worldviews and concepts you have been using to simplify your life. It can apprehend a new view and comprehend new ideas. Your ready understanding can bring together your experiences and scale them as vast to minute, animate to static, impersonal to intimate, and elaborate to simple. Your ready understanding will, when lifted by your wonder, take in the new.

Your ready understanding is intangible and yet forms the framework for tangible behaviors, and so has qualities of a built structure. To keep it from setting like cement, and so blocking your healing and cure, you can keep it up to date as you go. You can take apart your old understanding and craft a new and better one. In that way, as you note when your understanding is becoming obsolete, and you rework it to support your present processes of healing and cure, you are like Shiva, the deity that is a symbol of the destruction that is integral to creation.

Your ready understanding is open to dynamic realities that a rigid understanding would exclude. You can describe your ready understanding as flexible, expandable, and renewable. You can see it as able to take in things that are as small as your molecules of oxygen and as large as your ecosystem, that are as detailed as the pores of your skin or as nebulous as a distant galaxy.

Your ready perceptions allow you to see your dynamic body with the compassionate eye of an open and loving heart. With ready perceptions, you can look inside and out to find joys that heal and sorrows that weigh you down and divide you from a better future. With ready perceptions, you can approach harm with prepared forgiveness, and so make yourself free to retire harmful habits free of regret, shame, blame, or guilt and to form new habits of healing and cure that will change your life.

Ready perceptions open the door to loving all of the past that brought you to this moment of healing and cure, when you are choosing to create a better life than any you ever imagined. A ready heart shows the silver lining in each experience and the chances that are always arising all around you. A ready heart knows that you can see every moment and every event as a chance to become free of fear, to love self and others, to embrace change, and to look ahead with joy.

Ready perceptions are like an artesian well brimming over with sweet courage, delicious optimism, satisfying ingenuity, serene refreshment, and lively beauty that calls out your unique role in personal and shared healing and cure. Ready perceptions are the reading glasses through which you and you alone can see your healed body and your cured life.

Your ready sensations enable you to find things to support your states and habits of healing and cure. Your ready sensations include those that you remember; that prompt feelings of comfort, freedom, and happiness; and that may become guideposts, that is, that may mark your healing states and show you ways to discern, intensify, deepen, broaden, and extend those states.

Your ready sensations also alert you to events that require a prompt response. With hazards, your ready senses are like smoke detectors in an office building and your ready sense consciousnesses like the temperature at which its heat detectors activate the sprinklers. With finding your way, your ready senses are like onboard radar system and your ready sense consciousnesses are like patterns that show submerged shoals, rocky shores, and safe harbors.

Your ready energy arises from the channel that runs along the front of your spine and is centered below your navel. You can study it and alter it with the focus of your attention and concentration. As you heal, your dynamic body will become able to sustain the free flow of electromagnetic energy through the intangible structure of your subtle or energy body, that is, through its channels, centers, and meridians.

Ready energy prepares you to create and sustain healing states by adjusting the balance and flow of life energy. Ready energy thus flows freely through the intangible structures of your energy body and gives rise to fields that are strong at the core and decrease with distance. You can describe ready energy as strong, centered, calm, radiant, open, free flowing, and responsive. You can compare it with the water cycle of your bioregion, in which surface water flows downhill with gravity; fills low places like lakes and ponds; then, when it gets to the sea, evaporates to form clouds; and returns to the high places as snow or rain. That is, energy flows through and helps to form the landscape of your body.

Your readiness of energy is sapped by harmful states and habits that divert precious energy to poisonous states such as anger and to futile ones that form barriers. To ready energy, you can transform harmful states and habits, that is, divert their energy to states and habits of healing and cure. As you learn to do this, you are like the caretaker of a smart grid that sends electricity from areas of surge to those of lack to sustain flow and to prevent damage and waste.

Your ready flesh automatically syncs your biological processes, which are exquisitely complex, intricately interrelated, and dynamic. Ideally, your ready flesh includes a skeleton that is aligned to well support your organs; a nervous system that is calm, receptive, and responsive and also free of urges, irritability, or low spirits; an endocrine system that composes your metabolism; digestive and renal systems that allow nutrition and cleansing; a cardiorespiratory system that brings oxygen and removes waste; and so on.

Your fleshly systems are beyond the gateway of perceptions, and thus hide from awareness and understanding. Even so, you can learn to read their signals and, with the aid of experience and science, ready your flesh with needed foods, clean air and water, and other resources. When you do this, you are like a person who is living in a self-sufficient house and who tends its systems of water collection; food production; air and water purification; waste

29

processing, such as black water and composting; and the intake, production, and retention of energy.

When illness or injury interrupted your life, you may have lost the readiness of all or a part of your flesh and may have been using your time and attention to recover some readiness through surgery or the like. When you finish and are ready to return to sevenfold healing and cure, you can increase your readiness with common sense and by consulting doctors and writings.

As you do this you can take practical steps to avoid hazards such as viruses, impure water, and tainted soil; chemicals like formaldehyde, benzene, lead, alcohol, smoke, biocides, and so on; biohazards such as molds on poorly handled, sloppily prepared, or spoiled foods; and pollutants such as sulfur dioxide and biocides that irritate the immune system to cause problems such as asthma and food allergy.

You can also support your fleshly systems of healing and cure by avoiding adrenal overload due to overstimulation; by honing good daily habits such as modest exercise, sound sleep, and varied diet; and by forming and sharing healing states such as kindness and joy. You can also use a system of sevenfold healing that seeds processes of healing and cure that involve all levels of the body.

When your ready interbeing is in sync with time, you are not pulled back by the past or drawn into the future and thus can attend to healing and cure in the moment. To ready your interbeing, you can resolve your personal and shared time debts and begin to heal with life in time. When you have done this, you are already creating your new life and can focus on and trust in the here and now to seed the processes that will form your better, deeply fulfilling future.

With ready interbeing, every level of your body freely exchanges resources and processes that heal and cure your body as they heal and cure your region of the web of life in time. At the same time, all levels transform harmful states and habits and so help to heal all aspects of life in time. Your ready interbeing is like an accountant who keeps track of all that comes in and goes out and who keeps your expenses and savings up to date so that you can know your resources and use them as you choose.

When your interbeing is ready, you are at ease in time, that is, you are not stuck in the past or lost in fantasies about the future. You do not feel that you owe others or that they owe you. You do not take more than you give or use more than you replace. You live in balance with life in time and, as you heal, enhance rather than detract from the biosphere that generously provides for you.

Grounding

The modern paradigm grounds healing and cure in the tangible flesh and in what humans know of the flesh. Other paradigms ground healing in the earth, the web of life, or elsewhere. When you engage in sevenfold healing, you ground each level of the body in tangible features of flesh and interbeing and also in the intangible processes that join the core of your sevenfold body to the web of life and its matrix of space and time.

Your awareness is grounded at the top of your skull in the place where your soft spot was at birth. Thus, a part of your awareness is always resting in your flesh where it joins interbeing. From that point, your awareness can expand indefinitely and bring its focus to anything from the close, minute, and concrete to the distant, vast, and ethereal.

When awareness is ungrounded, it is like an untethered hot air balloon that may float away and be subject to gusts and shear forces, or get lost in fog, or run out of fuel, or descend abruptly and unexpectedly. When your awareness is grounded, your focus is tethered and can remain steady while moving to the inmost recesses of your flesh or to the edge of your known world. Your grounded awareness is thus like a communications tower that is fixed and can detect and tune into any signal in the multiverse. When your awareness is grounded, it becomes able to guide your understanding to apprehend and comprehend things.

Your understanding is grounded in your central nervous system, which includes your brain, spinal cord, and, for the purposes of

31

Sevenfold Healing Systems, the oft-neglected trunks of the autonomic nervous system that parallel your spinal cord. This view of the nervous system enables you to apprehend things by seeing patterns with the heart and gut as well as to know things through those parts of the brain that process language, vision, and shape.

Your understanding is also grounded in the body of knowledge that humans sustain in dynamic equilibrium with life in time. Moments of disequilibrium, as with "aha" moments of new apprehension or comprehension, may shift this body of knowledge. Now, at the end of the modern era, when understanding may be buried in heaps of data, you can enhance your grounding by taking time to discern and attend to what matters.

When your understanding is ungrounded, you may take anything as true and may make poor judgments that result in tragic mistakes or get lost in wishful thinking that wastes precious resources. If you do not ground your understanding, you are like the emperor who had no clothes and who was so deluded by self and others that only a fresh-eyed child could see the truth and say it aloud.

If your understanding is ungrounded, and you have authority over others, you may do great harm. You see this in leaders with strong, groundless ideas who persuade nations to act in ways that waste life and liberty. Thus, when your understanding is ungrounded, you are like the captain of a ship of fools who cannot use a compass or an anchor. By grounding your understanding in the human experience and in the core of your sevenfold body, you create the possibility of using both your compass and your anchor.

You can describe your grounded understanding as solid, sensible, prudent, earthy, and resilient as well as open to and inclusive of all learning. Your grounded understanding is thus like the ocean canoes in which the first Polynesians arrived in Hawaii, which held food crops and other fruits of a culture and which thus enabled those Polynesians to begin a new life in a new place and to live in their own way.

Your perceptions are grounded in your heart, which is the source of your sweetest and most treasured healing states and abilities and the crucible in which you can transform your harmful states and habits, including those complex habitual responses that seem to be as fixed as scars. Your grounded perceptions are also anchored in the hearts of all other sources of life that are near to you in space and time, and through them, to all others. Grounded perceptions thus arise from your heart and from all other hearts, each of which brings essential healing and cure to the web of life in time.

You can see your grounded perceptions as extending from your heart into the web formed by limitless numbers of hearts, each of which is a source of healing abilities such as altruism, compassion, joy, and equanimity. You can describe your grounded perceptions as loving, open, life affirming, fearless, forgiving, easy, or generous.

When you do not ground your perceptions, you may see your heart as loveless, your body as beyond healing, and your life as worthless. You may turn toward sickness and death, deepen your harmful states and habits, and develop new complex habitual responses that close off your heart and your interbeing. You may weaken your sevenfold grounding and divide your body from the abundant healing and cure of the web of life.

When your perceptions are not grounded in your core, you can describe them as heartless, weak, twisted, ugly, withered, or gray. When your perceptions are not grounded in interbeing you can describe them as nihilistic, depressing, toxic, worthless, or evil.

When you ground your perceptions, you become able to see the astonishing and boundless beauty in your body, in your life, and in your world. You can see and embrace your sanguine courage, abide in sweet healing states, and strengthen your healing habits and abilities. You can envision a new and better life and do what you need to do to bring it into being for the sake of self and others.

Your senses are grounded in your skin, that is, in your tangible flesh where it meets tangible interbeing. Your sense consciousnesses are grounded in the organs that read sensory data, such as your retinae and visual cortex, and in all your past readings of sensory data, such as images recorded in your memory. When you ground your senses in your tangible flesh and in tangible interbeing, you amass accurate data; when you ground your sense consciousnesses in past and present readings of those data, your sensations become available to you for use in sevenfold healing and cure.

When you do not ground your senses in the tangible, you may turn your sensations from healing to harming. For example, you can focus so intently on the baseline signal of your auditory nerve as to sense it as a ringing or a buzzing. In contrast, you may take the pain of a broken bone for that of a bruise. You may make like mistakes when you do not ground your sense consciousnesses in the full range of your past and present experience. For example, you may think that you hear a melody that you are only remembering or, like a child, imagine that you hear a monster talking in the closet. Your ungrounded sensations can thus mislead you and lead you to do great harm by spreading anxiety or disregarding hazards.

Your grounded sensations are like a thermometer and a record that you keep of the temperature and your body's impressions of it. Then, when your sevenfold body meets with a temperature that is new or unusual, you have a record of similar events that form the context for your present experience. To ground your sensations, you can transform harmful ones in the way of a teen who learns to transform the groundless fears of childhood into the mature habit of fearless prudence.

Your energy is grounded in your skeleton where it is in contact with the earth, that is, at the weight-bearing points where your flesh is in direct or indirect contact with bedrock. When seated, you ground your body through your sit bones; when walking, through the soles of your feet; and when lying prone, through your spine, pelvis, and heels. When outdoors, you ground your energy through direct contact with rock or through indirect contact via soil or trees. When indoors, you ground your energy through a floor, stair, or similar structure that rests on the solid earth beneath.

When your energy is ungrounded, you may feel that you can't settle, put down roots, land on your feet, or hold your ground. You may feel a nagging sense of being lost, disoriented, restless, or rootless, and may conceive of it as doubt, uncertainty, hesitancy, anxiety, insecurity, instability, skepticism, or discontent. When the distress is intense, your ungrounded energy is like a live wire that flails in all directions, propelled this way and that by surges of current that are seeking places of low charge.

Your grounded energy is like a shelter where you put aside cares, concerns, or distractions and feel strong, easy, and replete. When you ground your energy, you free yourself to attend to the practices that seed relief, wellbeing, transformation, and cure and to prepare to discern and realize your purpose in life.

> *Practice: Grounding Your Energy.* If you sense that your energy may be ungrounded, you can realize important healing by grounding it. To do so, you can assume a good posture and rest your awareness on your weight-bearing points, that is, on your sit bones when in a chair; your soles when walking; and your skull, spine, tailbone, and heels or soles when lying down.
>
> For example, you can sit on a firm chair with your knees bent at right angles; the soles of your feet resting flat on the floor; your spine erect and relaxed; your head tipped easily forward to allow for the free flow of spinal fluid; your sit bones in good contact with the seat beneath you; and your palms resting on your thighs.
>
> When you are set, take a few slow, deep breaths and allow your awareness to descend to your sit bones. To guide your focus, you can place your palms on your sacrum with your fingers touching in the midline, bring your focus to your palms, and allow your focus to descend to your seat. If need be, you can sit on your palms for a moment and so draw your awareness down to your sit bones.
>
> If you like, you can lie on your back instead of sitting down. Find a reasonably firm surface and pillows to support your

head and knees as needed and then lie down with your spine extended; your head tipped slightly forward; your palms resting on your pelvic bones; and the weight of your skull, spine, sacrum, and feet relaxing deeply into the surface below. You then take a few deep, slow breaths and bring your focus to your palms; then allow your focus to sink below your sacrum. If you like, you can place your palms under your sacrum to guide your awareness.

If you have difficulty creating or sustaining your grounding, you can try the seven-point posture of Vairocana or the Burmese posture for meditation, which can perfectly support your grounding and which you can learn from a teacher or from a media source that suits you. If you still have difficulty, you can work through the exercises in the *Manual* or find and consult a teacher of yoga or meditation. When you have learned to ground your energy body, and can move your focus at will, you will be able to ground your energy by bringing your focus into the central channel and moving it to a place several finger-widths below your navel.

Your flesh is grounded in the major organ systems that interface with interbeing, that is, in the organs of respiration, digestion, and excretion that nourish and that cleanse your flesh. In other words, your flesh is grounded in the lungs, kidneys, intestines, liver, and sweat glands that supply, sustain, and refresh your tissues.

Your flesh is also grounded in the matter, energy, and activities of interbeing, that is, in the matter that you exchange with streams, plants, animals, bacteria, and minerals; in the energy that combines with your matter as heat, sunlight, and so on; and in the processes of exchange that bring matter and energy in and return them to interbeing. Your flesh is also grounded in your microbiome, that is, in the five or so pounds of bacteria that coat your membranes and skin, where they protect you from infections and produce nutrients.

If you do not ground your flesh, you may lack one or more of the nutrients that you need or retain toxins that impair your flesh. When you are ungrounded, you may be like a person who is obese and yet malnourished, that is, who consumes empty calories that fail to nourish or to satisfy and so eats more and more and grows larger and larger without finding nourishment. Or, you may be like a person who eats organic foods that contain natural biocides such as mycotoxins or who eats conventional foods that contain biocides added through sprays or genetic engineering. These biocides may poison the flesh, enter into fat stores, and sicken the microbiome and so seed disease, disrupt the body's equilibrium, and undercut inborn systems of healing and cure.

You can ground your flesh by providing it with clean air, clean water, and well-tended, biocide-free foods that provide the matter and energy needed for your efficient and effective search for relief, wellbeing, transformation, and cure. When you ground your flesh in interbeing, it will automatically support your healing and cure. It will become like an infant who can grow and develop by eating when hungry and drinking when thirsty.

Your interbeing is grounded in every level of your sevenfold body and in the web of life in time, that is, in the larger interbeing created by all forms of life. Because interbeing is a relatively new concept, and because your part of it is neither static nor simple, you can ground your understanding of interbeing by taking time to think of it and to bring it into your worldview in a way that suits you.

> *Practice: Grounding Your Interbeing.* You can begin by thinking of every level of the body as reaching through your part of interbeing to find grounding in life in time. In your mind's eye, you can see this as myriads of invisible threads arising from each level of the body and extending out through your part of interbeing so as to interweave with the like threads that are arising from other generative sources of life. In this way you can see that your part of interbeing holds the dynamic links that ground each level of your body to all other forms of life in time.
>
> Looking more closely at the grounding of each level through your part of interbeing, you can see threads of awareness that represent processes of attention and concentration; threads of

understanding that symbolize processes of apprehension and comprehension; and threads of perceptions that show processes of compassion, altruism, and joy. You can then see threads of sensations along which matter and energy move to prompt a response, as when aromas scatter and stimulate appetite or when sound waves carry conversation. You can then see threads of energy transfer that join you with the world around, as when heat warms you and when energy exits your crown as outward awareness; your throat as speech; your navel as strength of purpose; and your root as creativity.

If you like, you can picture the threads that arise from your flesh on various scales, beginning with those that are microscopic. You can see RNA messages leave cell nuclei, hormones embrace membrane receptors, enzymes make proteins, neurons carry passing thoughts, oxygen enter from nearby plants, and soil bacteria refresh your microbiome. You can then see threads on a human scale, as when your lungs expand, your heart contracts, your kidneys purify your blood, your legs carry you to work, and all of your body cultivates good food. You can then see the threads on a vast scale, as when the strong and weak nuclear forces bind your atoms together and the sun's light travels across space to stimulate your pineal gland.

Up to this point, your image has been still. You can now allow it to become a moving image that starts at any time after conception and reveals your tangible and intangible interconnections with shared interbeing moving with your animate body and changing with the dynamic patterns of your daily life and your lifetime. As you do this, you can see your processes of becoming.

You can then see that to sync with life in time, you can put to rest and leave behind processes that belong in the past. In other words, you can resolve your time debts by paying or forgiving them. As you do this, you can conclude processes of your living past that hinder your healing and cure. These may have begun long ago and far away, as with warfare, domination, and use of fossil fuels, or recently and within you, as with blame of self or others for the interruption in your life. As you put the past to rest, you take care to note and keep processes that support your healing and cure, such as uplifting memories of joys or ease. You also begin to shape your legacy by adding processes that enrich the living present and that may enhance the living future.

In this picture, your part of interbeing holds the bonds of family, society, and culture, especially those that arise from all levels of the body. Your part of interbeing also holds the bonds that join you with other species, as with working animals, pets, and gardens as well as beloved habitats, wildernesses, and bioregions. As with all levels of the body, your part of interbeing also weaves you into the fabric of space and time.

When your part of interbeing is ungrounded, you may feel isolated or disconnected. You may feel as if you are standing at a crossroads and have no idea which way to go. Or, you may lack confidence in your surroundings or in your future, and so get lost in fantasies of a past golden age or a future paradise. You may lose your chance to be, to become, and to leave a legacy that realizes your life purpose.

When your part of interbeing is grounded, you are at ease with your surroundings and with your past and present, and the threads that connect you with the web of life in time are strong and resilient. To ground your part of interbeing, you can enhance your relations with other forms of life and with the here and now.

Relaxation

When your sevenfold body is ready and grounded on all levels, and you have caught up on sleep and nutrients, you are ready to relax. Because you are living in the post-industrial information age, you may tend to apprehend relaxation as ease and to comprehend it as the release of muscle tension or adrenal overstimulation. In other words, you may hold a narrow view of relaxation.

The reason that this narrow view is popular is that late modern habits of living tend to prompt certain states of sevenfold tension, as when prolonged sitting or standing and repetitive, rapid, detailed, or concurrent tasks lead to sustained tension in muscles. This form of tension also arises when you do tasks that you learned in relation to subtle or overt force and that are still linked to states of fear or duress. Modern habits may also prompt the perennial tension that can arise when habits are fixed rather than dynamic; are awkward rather than easy; or are linked with harm on one or more levels of the sevenfold body, as when you become aware that they may be unethical, pointless, wasteful, thoughtless, harmful, or immoral.

As you learn to recognize, to enter into, and to sustain sevenfold states of healing and cure, you will enhance ease and relaxation on all levels. Whereas some moderns may feign passing ease with harmful states of denial or harmful habits of drugs or thrills, you will become able to leave harmful states and habits behind for good and to embody the primordial states and habits that support inborn systems of healing and cure.

On the level of awareness, your relaxation creates a clear, smooth, intangible background in which you will be able to move your alert, easy focus of attention and concentration as you please and to rest it where you wish. Tibetan Buddhists learn this relaxation through a practice called shamatha, that is, tranquility meditation, in which your relaxed background of awareness is like a cloud-free sky and your relaxed focus of attention and concentration like a butterfly resting on a flower.

On the levels of understanding and perceptions, relaxation allows your mind to grow quiet, that is, to leave behind useless or harmful states and habits. When you relax on these levels, you may become aware of an astonishing number of useless and repetitive thoughts and of harmful states that are complex, intense, and recurring. When you transform such patterns, you will ease their grip and become able to relax into healing states and into new and familiar habits of healing and cure.

On the levels of sensations, flesh, and interbeing, your relaxation will enable you to withdraw attention from distractions such as background noise and from thoughts that prompt harmful states of anxiety, aggression, or craving. Likewise, relaxation will enable you to interrupt harmful habits such as cycles of pain in which muscular tension deepens pain, which deepens tension, and so on. You can also withdraw from processes that arise outside your body, as when you disengage from media that link you to distant sorrows that sap your resources by instilling harmful states, offering no way to ease or to redeem those states, and by diverting resources that you could use to further your intentions as you ease the harm that is in you or that is close to you.

On the level of energy, relaxation allows your resources to follow your intentions, that is, to flow away from processes that are useless or harmful and toward ones that support your healing and enable you to envision a new and better life. Put differently, relaxation of energy allows energy to flow from areas of waste to areas of need.

Focus

Your focus of attention and concentration enables you to know any part of the sevenfold body directly and thoroughly and to access and apply your intangible resources to its healing and cure. To prepare your focus for healing and cure, you relax it and strengthen it. As you do this, you are like an adult who learns to play the piano by first learning to move with ease and then to grow in strength and endurance.

To prepare your focus, you ensure that it is relaxed, that is, loose and light and effortless. If it is tight, burdensome, or strained, you are not ready to use it. Relaxing your focus may be difficult if your years in school formed your understanding at the expense of other levels of the body. For example, you may have learned to rely on harmful states of aggression or anxiety to focus and may have sustained your focus with harmful states of adrenal stimulation. If so, you may have become able to absorb large quantities of data in short periods of time and unable to learn from experience, to think

41

things through over time, or to hone your common sense through trial and error.

To relax your focus, you can withdraw your attention from habits that make you like a machine or a computer. As you do this, you direct that attention to your life—you can observe your life closely, think it through, note and transform harmful states and habits, and form new habits for a better life.

Once you have relaxed your focus, you can safely increase your concentration. You begin this slow and gradual process by letting your focus be soft and slight and by sustaining your relaxation as you allow your focus to grow narrower and more intense. You thus gently enhance the strength and endurance of your focus until you can sustain it with ease and rest it wherever you like. If you wish, you can support this with shamatha or insight meditation or with a complete set of practices for self-guided healing and cure.

On the level of awareness, you shift from the background to the foreground. As you do this, you are like a spectator who is part of the audience in a theater and who, as the lights go down, focuses on the curtain and then zooms in on the set, the action, the actors, and their telling expressions or gestures. As you practice sevenfold healing and cure, you remain aware of the audience as you do this, that is, you remain aware of the background of your healing, which is your body and your life.

You can thus describe the background of your awareness as open, empty, and expansive. You can see it as an unobstructed, unbounded backdrop that sets off the foreground. You can describe the foreground of your focused awareness as free, mobile, and easy and as ever stronger and more precise. As it develops, your focus is like a lens slowly and gradually zooming from a wide shot to a close up; a diffuse light narrowing into a spotlight; or the image of a camera obscura that becomes clearer as you move the film closer to the pinhole.

Your energy, flesh, and interbeing form the subtle structure that holds your focus. If your focus is like a spotlight, the other levels of the sevenfold body are like the grid on which the spotlight hangs. In other words, the other levels of the body allow your focus to go and to stay where you will. For example, when developing the healing ability of compassion, the other levels will help you to bring your focus to your heart, to a fleshly source of pain, or to another being that is ailing.

Your understanding, perceptions, and sensations can guide your focus. For example, they can pinpoint the complex habitual responses that prompt harmful states and habits so that you can observe and alter them, as by withdrawing the energy of attention from those that bar healing or cure. Likewise, these levels of the body can direct your focus to and thereby strengthen your healing states and habits. As you weaken barriers to healing and cure, all levels of your body combine to assist your focus as you deepen your healing and cure.

Strength

To support your healing states, you can enhance the strength of your sevenfold body, that is, the endurance and character that will enable you to seed and to sustain processes of healing and cure. You can think of this strength as that of a long-distance runner rather than like that of a weight lifter. To enhance this strength, you can develop abilities and habits that help you in the long haul, such as patience, persistence, practicality, and determination.

At the level of awareness, strength supports a relaxed background that is unimpeded and unbounded and a focus that is easy, steady, and suited to the scale and intensity of the task at hand. You can compare a strong background to an open countryside endowed with abundant fresh air and clean water; you can compare a strong foreground to a runner who flies over and enjoys the landscape while adjusting pace, route, and strategy.

At the levels of understanding, perceptions, and sensations, your strength increases with virtues that enable you to divert resources from harm to healing. Thus, a strong understanding, a brave and loving heart, and well-attuned sensations support you to detect and to sustain healing states and habits and to divert resources such as the energy of attention from harmful states to healing ones.

At the level of energy, you can increase your healing strength by drawing energy into your central channel and by enhancing its free flow through your central channel and chakras. Your strength can thus grow in proportion to your centering, your ease, and your vitality. Strength of energy is thus like the heat emitted from a steam radiator, which increases with pressure, flow, and degree.

At the level of flesh, strength derives from the mass of your muscles, bones, and other tissues, which may be lost with debility. Strength also derives from your vitality, which supports all levels of the sevenfold body. You can increase your strength with modest exercise such as walking and by easing harmful states and habits that waste or misuse resources. When you strengthen your flesh, you bring up inborn healing systems such as the immune system and enhance your ability to adapt to change.

At the level of interbeing, your strength grows with the number and depth of your ties to life in time. That is, the more ties you sustain with ease with plants, pets, friends, and family members, and the deeper those ties, the greater your strength of interbeing. Likewise, the strength of your interbeing increases as you allow your ties to extend over time into your community and your bioregion.

Resilience

Resilience is your sevenfold body's tendency to return to its baseline state or a more stable one of greater healing and to sustain the dynamic steadiness of its processes on all levels. In that way, resilience can be described as poise, balance, continuity, and evenness. By virtue of resilience, your life can become and remain steady and easy through interruptions and changes. Your resilience will grow as you heal and may enable you to stay steady through changes that are quick or abrupt.

On the level of awareness, resilience allows you to focus on what matters by allowing distractions to fade into the background. It lets you stay alert to new sources of harm and healing and to focus on them and assess them and, if need be, alter them. With resilient awareness, you can stay on task, that is, you can focus on a thing or on a series of things that matter to you. Your resilient awareness is thus like a radar scanner that filters out random scatter to reveal key landmarks.

On the level of understanding and perceptions, resilience lets you note when your experience is at odds with your expectations, find out why, and alter your understanding and perceptions to fit your reality. This resilience allows you to be responsive to events, to weather setbacks, and to adapt to the here and now, that is, to sync with life in time. With this resilience, you are like a student who uses life as a classroom in which life is the teacher and it leads you to form a dynamic worldview and to take fitting actions.

On the level of sensations and energy, resilience is your capacity to respond to extremes by enhancing signals that are too weak and by damping those that are too intense. In other words, it protects your sevenfold body from lack and from excess. When you develop this resilience, you are like an electrician who can boost weak circuits and add breakers that prevent burnout in the event of a surge.

On the tangible level of flesh and interbeing, your resilience is the tendency of your physiology to return to its usual state. In other words, each of your biological processes centers on an automatic set point that is like the setting of a thermostat. When you practice sevenfold healing and cure, you shift all of these set points toward healing and cure, which is like moving a team of jugglers down a gradual slope as they toss their clubs and balls back and forth.

Now, in the late modern era, when old and new toxins are filtering through the web of life into your body, your fleshly resilience to chemicals is of great importance. You may lack resilience if your liver is quick to form toxins, your fat is quick to store them, or your liver or kidneys are slow to remove them. You may also lack resilience if you take things in that tax your organs. With sound common sense, prudent trial and error, and savvy consultants, you can enhance your fleshly resilience by avoiding toxins and cofactors and by carefully cleansing your system.

45

On the intangible level of interbeing, your resilience lies in creating, sustaining, repairing, and enhancing your social and biological ties with life in time. By doing this in ways that are fun and easy for you, you ease the healing and cure of self and others.

Chapter 2. Habits for Healing

In the previous chapter, you prepared to enhance your state of being at any given moment in time by entering into a healing state, that is, by being healing. In this chapter, you prepare to deepen, broaden, and extend those healing states, that is, to become healing. You can do this by doing practices that seed processes of healing and cure that become second nature and that change your body.

To establish habits for healing change, you may need to take charge of your body in a new way. You may have entrusted its care to others through old habits such as obedient helplessness that came into you through media or life experience. For example, you may have entrusted a family member or authority figure with the welfare of your sevenfold body or you may have suddenly or slowly given up your authority and responsibility to insurance agents, managers, and others who have come to make your decisions for you.

You can take charge of your sevenfold body by choosing to guide your healing and cure, by taking on a daily formal healing practice, and by making careful choices as you access shared resources. These shared resources include complex systems such as clinics and hospitals; products like pills, elixirs, or devices; and processes such as medical advice, rituals, recipes, or ideas. Should any not further your healing and cure at this time, you can pass over them and return to them later time if and when you like.

Through your daily healing practice, you can learn formal exercises that seed and sustain processes that will aid your healing and cure in proportion to your time, effort, and wits. While your past education and experience may ease your way now if they helped you to form dedication, creativity, and character, they may also bar your way now if they instilled harmful habits of dependence, fear, or dislike. To open the way forward, you can rely on your strong and dynamic intentions as you form new habits of healing and cure that will transform your old habits of harm.

As you undertake a daily practice, you can set your intentions to learn how to guide your practice so as to enhance your inborn healing processes, transform harmful states and habits, retire useless ones, and work with consultants who can support your self-guided healing and cure. Because you will sync with life in time in order to become healing, you can use your daily practice to heal your ties with life in time.

Enhancement of Healing Habits

As you become familiar with your present habits, you see that life comprises processes of destruction as well as creation, that is, of harm as well as of healing. This means that you have habits of healing that you can discern and enhance. For example, you may note that you treat your flesh kindly and choose to strengthen that habit. Seeing the eternal nature of destruction and creation also enables you to note and to take in the healing habits of others. For example, you may be waiting in a lobby where the staff members are inept or unkind and you feel helpless to act; then you see and emulate a patient who talks to them with kind, clear insistence and thus shifts their processes of care toward competence and courtesy.

As you establish your daily practice of sevenfold healing, you can seed and sustain habits of healing and cure by using a complete series of practices like that in the *Manual*, which you can sample and play with below.

Practice: Healing Affirmations. When your life was interrupted by illness or injury, you may have lost your intentions or exhausted your kind compassion. Even after the first crisis passed, you may have continued to feel sad, disheartened, angry, or withdrawn. You or others may have further barred your recovery via complex habitual responses that entailed punishment, avoidance, or censure. To gently regain your authority over the sevenfold body, and to turn your perceptions to healing and cure, you can do a daily practice in which you select and repeat phrases to help your discern and enhance your relief and wellbeing.

To prepare, you set aside twenty minutes a day during which to do the exercise; you also identify a comfortable place in which to do it where you will be free of interruptions and distractions. The day before you practice, scan the groups of affirmations that follow below. Say aloud or silently any that appeals to you, see if it inspires relief or wellbeing and, if so, mark it in the book, jot it down, or remember it. As the day goes by, recall and repeat the phrase or phrases that you like best, playing with the wording and adding any new phrases of your own that you may prefer.

This body is returning to its original intent
This body is taking charge of itself
This body is centered here
The core of this body is gathering strength
The core of this body is resilient
The core of this body has authority over this body
The core of this body is responsible for this body
The authority that this body lost is returning
The responsibility that this body lost is returning now

This body is essential
This body is miraculous
This body is enough
This body is life and the living of it
This body is being and becoming healing

The core of this body responds to my wise care
The core of this body responds to the wise care of my doctors, counselors, and bodyworkers

This body is not a machine
This body is more than the sum of its molecules
This body is beyond human understanding
This body is more than my healing states
This body is more than my healing processes
This body is more than my healing practices
This body is more than my aware, alert, relaxed, grounded awareness

This body is more than my keen understanding
This body is more than my loving perceptions
This body is more than my sense connections
This body is more than my flowing life energy
This body is more than my miraculous flesh
This body is more than my part of interbeing
This body is more than the sum of its seven levels

This body can love this body
This body can guide this body
This body can care for this body
This body can heal this body
This body can cure this body
No one can care for this body as I can
No one can know this body as I can
No one can love this body as I can
No one can heal this body as I can
No one can cure this body as I can

This body is a precious gift
This body is mine to love and care for
This body is part of the web of life
The web of life is healing this body every moment
The web of life is nourishing this body every moment
The web of life is sufficient
The web of life is essential to me
I am essential to the web of life
All healing centered outside me heals me
All healing centered within me heals others

Those who love me are healing me
I am healing those I love
Healing is everywhere
Any harmful process can become a healing one
I will be able to turn this harm into healing
Loss is a natural part of this life
Death is the natural end of this life
Death is a reminder to embrace this life

I can make the most of each moment
I can make the best of each moment
I can make good on each moment
I can turn harming into healing
I can take loss as a chance for new life
I can discern and take wise advice
I can find consultants who can help me
I can heal with others
I can heal with the web of life

When practice time comes, take this book and a notepad and pencil and go to the place you chose. Then prepare your sevenfold body as noted in *Part Two, Chapter 1* above, that is, by ensuring good posture, grounding, relaxation, and so on. When you are ready, relax your eyelids and invite deeper relaxation by taking several slow, deep breaths. As you do this, visualize your breath letting in healing light and letting out darkness and ill being.

Now write down one to ten phrases you would like to use during this practice session. Favor any that increase your feelings of relief or wellbeing at the present moment. To support your memory, write out the phrases on your notepad and then repeat them slowly and easily for ten minutes, pausing to enjoy relief and wellbeing as they arise. When your time is up, offer thanks for this chance to practice and share your healing with others by picturing yourself accepting relief and wellbeing with them. As you finish, take a few minutes to discern your state. If your state feels like a healing one, enjoy it as long as you like.

If you feel that the phrases are not quite right for you now, you can devote one or more practices to trying out a variety of phrases so as to find those that best support your ongoing processes of healing and to become familiar with your present healing states.

Practice: Aloha Breathing. After setting aside a week in which to learn this new Hawaiian practice, you can make free use of it whenever and wherever you like. Aloha breathing uses a visualization to join the energy of breathing with that of awareness. You can prepare for it by finding a place to sit in a good posture like that described in

Part Two, Chapter 1, that is, with your feet flat on the floor or ground, your ankles and knees at right angles, your sit bones planted firmly on your seat, your head tipped slightly forward, and your spine straight and relaxed and ready to support your lungs as they fill and empty freely, fully, and easily.

When practice time comes, assume your good posture and rest your palms over your sacrum with the tips of your outer fingers touching at the midline. Now, bring your awareness to the crown of your head in the place where your soft spot, or fontanelle, was at birth. When your awareness is resting easily, allow it to descend to your neck, and then gradually down your spine to your pelvis, where you bring it to your sacrum beneath your palms. Gently allow your focus to fall slowly to your sit bones, and then down your leg bones to the soles of your feet. When your awareness is resting on your soles, take several slow, deep, cleansing breaths in which you allow in healing light and allow out the darkness of harm.

Now, at the end of your final cleansing breath, gently push all of the air out of your lungs until they are completely empty and then, without pausing on the out breath, begin to breathe in slowly until your lungs fill completely. As you breathe in, sweep the focus of your attention up through your leg bones, pelvis, and spine to your crown and on up above your head, where you visualize your breath forming an intangible tree that rises from your crown. Allow the tree to be as small or as large as suits your breath.

At the end of the in breath, pause briefly with your lungs full of air and imagine that you are taking shelter under the canopy of your intangible tree. When you are ready, breathe out slowly. As you breath out, sweep the focus of your awareness back down through your skull, spine, pelvis, and leg bones to the soles of your feet. When your lungs are completely empty, begin another cycle without pausing. Continue the cycle of breathing and visualizing the tree until you are able to do it with ease.

When the focus of your attention is moving easily with your breath, add the word aloha. That is, as you begin your in breath, you form the syllable "ah" in your throat and allow your in breath to form the sound rather than forming it with your vocal cords. Then half way through the in breath, let the flow of your breath form the syllable "loh" and allow it to taper off as you reach the end of the in breath and visualize the tree. As you breathe out, allow your breath to form the syllable "hah." You then continue the cycle of breathing, visualizing, and aloha until you are doing it with ease.

You then add a healing idea of the word aloha. You can think of it as "welcome," that is, as a greeting that expresses easy-going, delighted, kind connection. Or you can think of it as "breath of God," that is, as relaxing into easy participation in the renewal of spirit through breath. If you like, you can also imagine that you are receiving the sacred gift of a Hawaiian flower lei.

When you have become comfortable with the full practice, you can repeat it ten times or as many times as you like. When you finish, note the connection you are forming between the earth beneath your feet, your body, and a heavenly place above your crown. Note and enjoy the intangible sevenfold alignment and integration that are enhancing with this practice.

If you like, use aloha breathing whenever you like for refreshment, as when you are distracted, pulled in many directions, or dissociated from your surroundings. Use it also to enhance your healing state and, if it suits you, to wind down or to go to sleep.

Transformation of Harmful States and Habits

As you deepen your direct knowing of the sevenfold body, you will find that harmful states and habits are weakening your body by stealing precious resources, such as the energy of attention, from your ongoing processes of healing and creation. For example, you may note a pattern of malicious thought or gossip that you can transform by turning your attention to affirmations or aloha breathing and thereby restore your healing states, habits, and abilities.

Chances are good that you will find that many of your harmful states and habits were formed early in life, before you were able to apprehend or comprehend anything and when you absorbed the habits of those around you at an astonishing rate. You became so used to these harmful states and habits that you never realized they were not serving you well. Later, after you began to apprehend patterns and to comprehend concepts, you continued to establish harmful states and habits without seeing the harm in them and thus accumulated a storehouse of burdensome states and habits.

To recover the resources that your harmful states and habits are diverting from your healing and cure, you can observe them as they arise and note those that do the most to undermine your healing states and habits. You can then change one, and then the next, and the next, and so on until you renew the way you are in the world. You can change as shown in the ancient symbol of the enneagram, in which the youthful habits that hold you back become the ones that change so as to define your maturity.

The practices that transform your harmful states and habits are esoteric. That is, they seed meditative and practical processes that yield new insights and perspectives and thus enable you to create healing changes inside and out. Depending on the harmful state or habit in particular and its links to your living past, the changes may be simple or complex, happy or harrowing.

For example, if a harmful habit is formed by chance, and is not linked with intense states of being, you may find it easy to transform. If, in contrast, it forms a thread through your living past, or came into you linked with force or duress, you may find it hard to change and may wish to take the change in many small or slow steps. However you approach the esoteric work, it will be worth your while, and may yield joys beyond your present imagining. To get a taste of this work, you can play with the exercise below.

Practice: Response to Media. When you participate in media, they may assail your sevenfold body with memes that slip past your awareness and seed habits that are harmful, invasive, or addictive. With overuse of screens and multimedia especially, you may soon find that you have lost the ability to use media wisely. By taking the time and trouble to form healing habits, you can learn to use media selectively and, eventually, to turn any source of harm into one of healing and cure.

To begin, you can observe your complex habitual responses to various types of media and then take a media holiday that is like an elimination diet. When your media responses have become less set, you add back media that support your healing states and habits. Later, as you become better able to transform your responses, you add back more media. By following the instructions below, you can free yourself to use media by choice and so to sustain your ongoing processes of healing and cure.

> *Step One.* To prepare for step one, you choose and prepare two samples of visual media, one of which will prompt in you a strongly negative response and the other of which will prompt a strongly positive one. If you like, you can set aside two books of photographs, or a DVD player and two time-coded DVDs on which you can readily access clips, or a laptop computer with a browser bookmarked to access two clips for online streaming. Whatever you choose, prepare the media so that you can watch it without listening to any audio, as when you mute any sound. Then, set aside half an hour of your daily healing practice during which you will be able to watch the media and to observe your responses.

> When the time comes for your practice, assume a comfortable posture, and begin by taking stock of each level of the sevenfold body. Begin by using your focus to note the contraction or expansion of your awareness; the thoughts that are arising in your understanding; the emotions that are alive in your perceptions; the dullness or acuity of your sensations; and the grounding of your energy body. When you assess your flesh, sweep your focus through your body from your crown to your soles and back again. When you assess your part of interbeing, note your present feelings about your past, present, and future surroundings. Discern whether you are in a harmful state, that is, whether you have lost relief or wellbeing. If so, take a few slow deep cleansing breaths to each your sevenfold body.

Note: If you have difficulty bringing the focus of your awareness to your pelvis to assess your grounding, you can guide your focus by placing your palms over your sacrum with your fingertips touching lightly in the midline. If you prefer, you can cup one hand over your tailbone or sit briefly on your palms.

Now access the media clip that will prompt your negative response. Verify that the sound is off and then watch the clip for one minute. Stop the clip and take stock of each level of your sevenfold body from awareness to interbeing. If your response to the clip abates as you observe your body, watch it again as needed to refresh your harmful state before continuing. Take special note of the state of your interbeing, that is, your sense of connection or disconnection with the people, plants, animals, and bioregions as well as with space and time. Observe your harmful state closely so that you will be able to recognize it when it arises in the future.

Now, watch the clip again to return to the harmful state and take stock of your body again. This time, guide your focus with your palm by placing it over your crown and then over your throat, heart, gut, navel, and lower belly. Each time you place your palm, take note of the emotions and fleshly sensations that belong to the harmful state prompted by the clip, using the media to restore the harmful state as needed. When you have finished, return your palms to your thighs and run your awareness from your crown down through your muscles and bones to the soles of your feet, taking care to note any emotions and sensations that you may have missed. Now take a minute to deepen your familiarity with this harmful state.

Now, take a few minutes to recall other times when you were in this state. Trace your memories back as far as they will go. If you are ready to do so, recall the first time you felt this way. As you explore the personal history of this state of being, take note of the thoughts, feelings, and memories that you associate with this state.

Note: If at any point in the exercise you encounter a living memory that is traumatic and that may prompt a response that may do extreme harm, as with freezing, dissociation, or aggression, place your hands on your thighs, bring your awareness to your weight-bearing points, and breathe slowly and deeply until the response eases. If you like, use aloha breathing to support your recovery. Then stop the exercise for the day and make a note of what you have learned about your personal history with this harmful state and any related habits of harm.

When you have become familiar with this harmful state, take time to recover. Begin with several slow, deep, cleansing breaths in which you let in healing light and let out all harm. If you like, use the aloha breathing for as many cycles as you wish. When you have released the harmful state, repeat the full exercise for the positive medium and for the healing state that it induces. When you finish, take time to enjoy the healing state and to become familiar with it. Note your relief and wellbeing and take it as a start point for your healing and cure. Prepare your expectations to reach deeper states of healing as you learn to create states that are strong and that you will be able to share with ease.

If you like, you can play with this method over the next week of daily practice sessions by choosing other clips that bring on clear states of harm or healing or that bring on complex states in which healing and harm coexist. As you do this, allow your awareness and understanding to illuminate the habits of harm and healing that are alive in you and that belong to your habits of response.

Step Two. When you have become familiar with your responses to media, take a media holiday. Do this for at least a week. If feasible, extend it to a month or a year. The idea is to take enough time away to be able to gain a new perspective on your response to and use of media, which you may miss out on if your holiday is too short.

If you use media in relation to your work, you can limit your holiday to times when you are not working. If you rely on certain types of information that you obtained through media in the past, pinpoint what you need to know and find a way to get it. For example, if you need to know the weather to plan your day, you may be able to ask a family member or to access a weather map that gives you the data you need and no more. Likewise, you may be able to keep up with social groups by talking with a friend. If you are addicted to certain media or to your responses to them, taper your use or go "cold turkey." You will know which is best for you.

On any rare occasions during your media holiday when you cannot avoid media, as when you are in a public place where a television is blaring, take note of the content and your response and consider whether your holiday has been long enough. Again, you will know what is best for you as you return authority and responsibility to your body and increase your health and happiness.

Step Three. When you finish your media holiday, set aside an hour a week in which to use media that are likely to prompt a healing state in you. You can choose those specifically intended for healing or cure or choose them based on your gut feeling as to what may help to heal or cure you in the moment.

When you have taught yourself to select media that support your sevenfold healing and cure, you can increase your media use at will. If at any time you sense that a medium is using you rather than the other way around, you can return to your media holiday and refresh your perspective and your ability to use media for healing and cure.

Step Four. In this step, you begin to transform your responses. The ultimate objective is to become able to use any medium to further your healing or cure and, eventually, to meet any life experience in the same way.

You can prepare for this exercise by thinking about how to use working questions, such as those below, in daily life. You do this by becoming familiar with a question or with a series of questions and then keep them at the back of your mind as you go about your day. When they come to mind, or a suitable moment arises, you can bring them to mind right away and think about them in the context of experience. In this exercise, you bring them to mind when you engage media and, if you like, when you note the unexpected or when your habits lead to poor results.

You also prepare for this exercise by becoming aware of common patterns in media, such as television programming that offers fraught content and is likely to prompt anxiety and helplessness. This programming leads into ads that relieve those feelings, usually by promising escape, indulgence, success, approval, or security. You can also prepare by noting the meditative nature of media watching, through which you may absorb the habits shown or held by commentators, actors, and characters.

Note: In the practice of sevenfold healing, you avoid desensitization, which is exchanging one harmful state for another. For example, with desensitization you watch media that prompt harmful states, such as fear, and transform them into other states, such as contempt. Because both fear and contempt are harmful states of aversion, you may seem to gain healing or cure but are in fact only concealing your harmful state from your awareness.

When you begin this exercise in daily life, you keep the working questions in your mind over the course of a week during which you observe media and your responses to it.

  a.   How am I responding to this content right now?
  b.   What do I gain through this response? What do I lose?
  c.   Why do I respond like this?
  d.   How would I respond if I were healed or cured?
  e.   How do I wish to respond right now?

As you work with the questions, you are seeking to observe media that prompt healing states or mildly harmful states or habits. If you mistakenly engage media that have strong harmful effects, withdraw your attention immediately and refresh your state of being with cleansing breaths or aloha breathing.

If you respond to media with healing states and habits, feel free to enjoy that healing as you consider the working questions. If you respond with mildly harmful states or habits, stop and carefully consider the working questions. When you have weighed each one of the questions, look more deeply into your responses. See if you can get to the bottom of the living past that is responding to the media as if to protect your body from pain, to satisfy a craving, or to numb your feelings. As in *Step One*, look to pinpoint the original source of your response and the way that it lives on in you.

When the working questions reveal the source of an unnecessary state of harm, devise a way to ease that source so as to be able to use its energy for healing and free your body to leave it behind without effort or regret. If you have difficulty, you can consult a counselor or work through the complete set of exercises in the *Manual*.

Ideally, you free the energy trapped by the state of harm by forming healing habits such as noting the suffering of others and responding with spontaneous compassion; avoiding or taking prudent action to ease others who are trapped in states of harm; and responding with processes of healing or cure rather than with the harmful responses that arise when you sustain the weaknesses of your living past.

With experience, you will develop perspective and insight and will become able to draw on the healing abilities of the web of life in space and time and thus, over time, to transform any and all of your harmful responses into healing ones.

Retirement of Useless Habits

Many habits outlive their use, especially those that become second nature. Those that do not do active harm may persist unnoticed and accumulate, thereby sapping valuable resources from your processes of healing and cure. For example, you may ignore people whom you encounter every day because you are caught up in idle daydreams or are brooding on pointless dislikes. You thus waste energy and, at the same time, lose a precious chance to enhance your healing and cure by enjoying the people you see. To retire the useless habit of ignoring others, you can substitute a healing one such as that described here.

Well Wishing. You can offer well wishes at any time when you are surrounded by sources of life, as when you are sitting in a crowded room or walking in nature. If you rarely get outside, you can engage in well wishing while looking out a window, riding in a vehicle, or visiting a consultant.

When you notice a person, tree, blade of grass, flower, bird, insect, or any other source of life that you could enjoy but would usually ignore, you can remember that all living things embody processes of destruction and creation, that is, harm and healing, and that you can enjoy and share in their processes of creation. You silently support their processes of creation by offering well wishes such as: *May you be healed, May you be cured, May you thrive.* As you do this, allow your sevenfold body to remain relaxed, grounded, and easy, and enjoy each good wish as you offer it. If you like, you can vary your good wish, or blessing, to suit the circumstances.

If your attention wanders or is interrupted, you can gently return it to the sources of life around you and to your good wishes. If you are feeling run down at the time of your practice, you can offer some or all of the well wishes to yourself and can repeat them as often as you like. By doing and enjoying this practice often, you can make it a habit that is second nature and thus integral to your being, becoming, and interbeing.

Consultation with Counselors and Bodyworkers

Chances are good that you will consult one or more carers who have dedicated their lives to the study and practice of healing or cure. While they cannot do healing or cure for you, they may save you time, alert you to new sources of healing or cure, and give you access to shared services and to complex systems of care.

In sevenfold healing, a bodyworker can help you learn to recognize, enter into, and sustain healing states of being. When you look for a bodyworker, that is, a healer who works directly through the laying on of hands, you can seek out one who is ethical, kind, and certified in an ancient or modern method such as physical therapy, healing touch, deep tissue massage, chiropractic, Rubenfeld Synergy Work, accutonics, lomi lomi, craniosacral massage, or Reiki. Because bodywork is direct, personal, interpersonal, and expensive, and may help you most at the beginning of your healing, you can choose a bodyworker who is a well respected and try a session to find out if the consultant's hands are healing for you. If so, you can ask the consultant to help you learn to recognize healing states so that you will be able to recreate them on your own later one. If your flesh is sensitive, you can request a gentle form such as healing touch, Reiki, or craniosacral massage. If you face further obstacles, you can return to the bodyworker and ask for additional support.

In sevenfold healing, counselors are well-rounded psychologists, clergy members, or other experienced, qualified therapists who have weakened and dissolved their harmful states and habits and who may therefore be able to help you to do the same. As with finding a bodyworker, finding a counselor is personal. If you are struggling to transform your harmful states and habits, you can find a promising counselor and try a session to find out if the counselor is right for you. If not, you can keep looking. Ideally, you find one who can sustain an open awareness with a strong understanding, warm perceptions, and experience of inner work. One who has developed strong healing states and habits may be able to share them with you and offer useful, practical advice on how you might best become able to move toward healing and cure.

In sevenfold healing, doctors are practitioners of global mainstream medicine who have access to shared services such as hospitals and laboratories. That is, a doctor is licensed, fully qualified, well trained, experienced, and able to advise you on the latest science and technology. (*See Chapter 4 below for ideas to try when consulting with your doctors.*)

Chapter 3. Healing Abilities

When your life was interrupted by illness or injury, you may have found that you lost some of the abilities on which you relied and that others had become weak. In sevenfold healing and cure, you develop the abilities that you have at present, including those that may have been dormant, and apply them to your practices and processes of healing and cure. As you do this, you enhance those that support your healing and cure so as to make them second nature, that is, integral to your being and becoming.

As you advance, your healing abilities grow until you can open the gateway of your perceptions, admit anything without exclusion, and transform any harm into healing or cure. A key ability that can ease any other ability is right effort, that is, using a degree of effort that is poised between slacking and delay, on the one hand, and striving and hurry on the other. You can describe right effort as moving with the river of life rather than trying to push or to pull it. As you prepare to develop your inborn healing abilities, you can reflect on the ones described below.

Self-Guidance

To guide your healing and cure or, rather, to recognize that you are already guiding your own healing and cure and to take charge of them, you can set strong, resilient intentions. These can motivate your progress and join your processes of being and becoming to your goal of creating a new, fulfilling, and better life. You can then adjust your intentions on a regular basis to reflect your progress in healing and cure.

To visualize the adjustment of your intentions, you can imagine that you are a voyageur in a new world who is heading toward a distant mountain range. You can then see the terrain in between as a series of obstacles that you address one at a time, always keeping in mind your distant goal and what you can see of the obstacles ahead. Because the way ahead is unknown, and you know your location and your destination, you set intentions that will guide you from now on and that you can adjust to suit what you learn of the terrain just ahead. As you do this, you can call on abilities such as curiosity and ingenuity. When you have gained experience, you become a pathfinder, that is, you come into sync with life and time by way of dynamic and resilient intentions that develop as you go.

You can also think of self-guidance as the series of steps that you might take if you learned that you had pre-diabetes and aimed to limit your blood sugars levels so as to protect your blood vessels and organs. When you learn that your blood sugar is high, you eat well and do modest exercise until you lose fat. Your doctor finds that your blood sugar levels have returned to normal and does not advise pills or insulin. You keep to the diet and exercise and hold your weight steady. Your blood sugar levels remain normal. Some years later, your doctor finds that your blood glucose is high again. This time, your regimen does not bring it down. You consult with your doctor and choose to take pills. These work for a decade. After, when your blood sugar levels rise again, you consult with your doctor and choose to take insulin. You continue to take good care of your flesh as it changes.

In self-guided sevenfold healing, you can support your dynamic intentions by allowing them to reflect your ongoing life experience. You can do that by observing your states of being, your practices and processes of harm and healing, and your present situation. You can then adjust your expectations so that they are realistic as well as optimistic. This dynamism will allow you to pass with relative ease through times of trial and change as you hone your ability to realize your intentions through self-guidance; it is especially useful if your healing and cure are uncertain or confusing.

For example, you may be like someone who has multiple sclerosis and whose healing states and habits grow weak at certain times of day. You may note that at those times of day your symptoms, signs, and errors increase. To ease your difficulties, you can try taking a daily afternoon siesta. When you do, you find that the nap or rest eases your difficulties at other times of day and also enhances your abilities at those times. As you consult your doctors and adjust your treatments, you can experiment with regimens that you initiate to refresh your body and to be at your best whenever you can.

Likewise, if you tend to lose your abilities in the aftermath of a cold or flu, you can substitute a comfort practice for your daily formal healing practice during your recovery. That is, you can find relief by trying a hot pack or a cold pack, cuddling up with a favorite pillow and book, listening to relaxing music, consulting a bodyworker, or conducting a refreshing practice of meditation, Qi Gong, centering prayer, zikr, or chair yoga.

As part of healing with life in time, you can learn to recognize the present moment as one point in the moving currents of history that came into you in your first moments, that even now pass through you or live on in you, and that will, after your chance or deliberate transformation, live on as your legacy. By noting your place in the web of life in time, you can gain perspectives from which to see the healing that is always arising in self and others and to view the way ahead to your ultimate purpose. This big picture view can thus enable you to select your present practices and processes of healing and cure to suit your ultimate, realistic goals.

Self-guidance is the key to working well with consultants over time. As you get to know them, and to know your present system of medical care, you can observe what works and what does not. You can use life experience to hone your common sense, to guide your use of resources, and to stay open to new possibilities. As you do this, you learn to take advice that is good for you and to decline advice that is not.

When you view your healing and cure in the context of life in time, you can view the interruptions in your life as rites of passage that you pass through to come into sync with life in time and to heal and cure your life from now on. Then, you need not see the gaps in your life as abnormal, temporary, or wasteful; you can see them as belonging to the healing and cure of life in time and your part in them as your best chance to be and become healing and cure.

To take charge of your healing transformation, you can become aware of your state of being, discern and ease its fluctuations, and gauge and enhance your being and becoming. Because the dynamic processes of life are subtle as well as gross, and tangible as well as intangible, and because so many are automatic, you may find that it takes some time to become fully aware of your state of being and to learn how to shift it nearer to healing.

When you guide yourself, you become like Mark Twain when he was a steamboat pilot on the Mississippi River; as he made his way to a distant port, he and his crew used their intimate knowledge of the river to anticipate hazards and to take soundings to guide the boat through shifting sandbars. To use Sevenfold Healing Systems to support you in guiding yourself, you can use practices like those in *Part Two, Chapter 2* above or the complete set in *the Manual*.

Ways to Heal with Life in Time

Like springs of sweet water, your compassion, joy, and altruism rise from your center and, when ready, overflow into the ocean of life. Your purest healing abilities thus refresh your sevenfold being and becoming before going on to refresh interbeing. Likewise, the purest healing abilities of others refresh their bodies and then, if they are strong and you are open, they may refresh you.

Compassion. Compassion is the inborn tendency of your sevenfold body, especially your physical heart and perceptions, to recognize and respond to the suffering of others with sympathy. Compassion is not empathy, that is, you do not share a harmful state of pain or suffering; nor is it pity, that is, you do not engage in subtle or covert forms of triumph or punishment. When your compassion rises, you remain in a strong healing state aided by energy that is centered and balanced and respond with sympathy that is like an antidote to suffering as well as a call to eliminate it. Tibetan Buddhists describe compassion as a fine quiver of the heart, that is, a way of feeling with others that eases suffering rather than adds to it.

When you respond to suffering with harmful states or habits, you undermine your compassion and your other healing abilities and

65

hinder your being and becoming. When your healing states and habits are stronger than your harmful ones, you will be able respond to suffering with compassion that supports your sevenfold healing and cure even as it extends outward through your part of interbeing to ease the distress of others.

You can learn to express compassion as a flow of energy from self to others. When you offer compassion through healing touch or Reiki, you may be able to sense the life energy that flows in through your crown, down through your flesh, and out through your palms and soles. You may be able to feel it filling areas of lack in your sevenfold body and, as it flows into others, filling areas of lack in their bodies as well. If you like, you can note when your heart center is weak or aching and can place your palms on your breastbone. As you allow the energy of compassion to flow into your heart, you may feel your palms grow warm and your lack ease.

When your compassion is strong, you can share the energy of compassion without sapping your energy or limiting your healing states or processes. You may even note that the energy of your compassion, like that of any love, increases with the giving and flows to places of lack in self as well as in others. That is, you may heal yourself as you heal others and support healing and cure and being and becoming wherever the need is greatest.

When you respond to suffering with compassion, it is as if you are the happy new parent of your sevenfold body who loves it just as it is and who responds to its suffering with tender, brave hope and care free of doubts or boundaries. And, as you hold and treasure the infancy of your new and better life, you see that its wellbeing is one with all other precious sources of life and begin to feel with them and to respond to them as to your new self.

Joy. Joy is the sweetest shared healing state and the third of what Buddhists call the heavenly abodes. Like the healing states of altruism, compassion, and equanimity, the healing state of joy is a kind of love that nurtures your processes of being and becoming. When you can rest in joy at will, you will be able to see, to share in, and to enhance the healing and cure that are always arising in life

66

and time and that can inspire the bliss that is one with cure.

You can know joy from a centered healing state in which you note moments that seem absurd, new, or unexpected, and you can freely and playfully delight in them. You can nurture and enhance joy by noting and savoring sweet moments in which its fleeting love wells up in you, buoys your state of being, and overflows into life in time. You can invite joy by being always ready to share in the kind and ready laughter that lifts all processes of healing and cure.

Your joy can grow without limits when you are able to see and to share in the joy of others. This may come as second nature to you or may be long in coming. Whatever time and effort it takes you to respond with joy to the joy of others will be worth your while; you will discover and delight in the never-ending sources of joy around you. As you do this, you become a link in the chains of healing, loving joy that arise from and pass through all sources of life and that help to make life in time a limitless source of healing and cure.

Joy is thus like the stars of evening; yours is like the first star you see at dusk and that of others is like the Milky Way that spreads across the sky when the darkness is deepest and includes so many stars that you could not possibly count them in a lifetime. Joy is also like the stars of the universe, which form all sources of light in the history of life in time and which transform but never end. By responding with joy to the joy of others, you are like a stargazer who takes every light in the history of space and time as a personal source of personal healing and cure that you share with all.

When you respond to your life and to the lives of others with joy, you are like a sick person who has realized with delight that you will be healed and cured because healing and cure are always arising in every source of life. You can then open to the joy that is always in everyone, even when it has become dim, or is deeply hidden, or is barred by hazardous states and habits. You can bask in the light of creation that is all things, including the densest matter.

Altruism. Altruism is the love that knows no boundaries of matter or energy. In other words, it is love that is all-inclusive and never-ending. Altruism rises from the depths of your healing states and lights your face with a glow like no other. Your altruism is always available for healing but is easily drained or hidden by harmful or useless states or habits. When your being is clear, centered, strong, grounded, and alive with your other healing abilities your altruism can become strong. When it is strong enough to fill your being and to overflow into interbeing, it will carry all forms of love to all beings. Because altruism knows no favorites, it flourishes free of all harm, including that of power, control, preference, and agenda.

You can enhance your altruism by recalling and reliving it and by emulating it when you see it. For example, you may be able to recall feeling altruism when a wise elder or teacher showered love on you and left an indelible imprint of abundant earthy love. Or, you may be able to join with those who have the habit of offering well wishes, blessings, or prayers to all sources of life including those they will never see or know. Or, you may be able to emulate sages and prophets whose healing love knew no bounds or boundaries and whose present-day followers keep that love alive.

You can strengthen your altruism for the sake of self and others by using affirmations like those in *Part Two, Chapter 2*; by transforming personal and shared states and habits of harm; by leaving behind useless habits; by practicing metta meditation or following the path of blessing; by visualizing the pure heart light of every being you encounter; and by gently and resiliently loving your sevenfold body and interbeing with kindness, compassion, insight, perspective, grounding, and strength.

When you are in the healing state of altruism, you are like an elderly person whose friends and family have died and who has come to terms with sickness and mortality, who is no longer holding back or barring anything, and who can now see and enjoy the true worth of each form taken by the one life that holds all life.

Transformation of Harm

When your life is interrupted, you can greatly ease your healing and cure by noting and transforming harmful states and habits that waste time and sap energy. Because the harm that has lived in you longest will be doing you the most harm, and will have become a part of the background of your life, you may not be able to see it or may even assume that it is natural or needed. To transform this living past, you first gain insights and perspectives that reveal it.

To discern intangible sources of harm, you can do inner work like that in the exercises in *Part Two, Chapter Two* above or in the *Manual*, or you can consult a counselor or keep a journal. As you begin to see your harmful states and habits, and to get to the bottom of them, you can address any hidden lack they sustain and then withdraw the energy of your attention and turn it to your ongoing processes of healing and cure. In other words, you can reclaim resources that are working against you and engage them in working for you.

To discern tangible but unseen sources of harm, you can note that your flesh and interbeing are always taking in, digesting, and transforming biocides and other toxins. For example, your cells and your microbiome are breaking down myriads of compounds that would, if they built up, do passing or lasting harm to your tangible flesh and interbeing. To prevent this, your flesh breaks down toxins and your blood takes them from your tissues to your kidneys and liver for removal as waste. To support these ongoing processes of transformation, you can avoid toxins and refresh your tissues by drinking plenty of clean water or organic green or black tea.

Likewise, any bodily activity may do some harm, as when you hold habits of moving that are awkward and lead to tension or arthritis. You can prevent this by taking a Feldenkrais or yoga class that enables you to move more smoothly. Or you may note that you have too much body fat. When you look deeply into it, you may find that you were eating to ease old fears and then formed a cycle of hypoglycemia, in which you ate sugar, reached a blood sugar peak that led to a trough, which you eased by eating more sugar that remains as fat. You may then be able to break the cycle and release the fat that could become a reservoir for toxins.

When you have learned to move smoothly, or to release the fat that may harm you now or in the future, you can recover the energy of your attention and return it to your states and habits of healing and cure. As you return more and more energy to healing and cure, you become better able to see underlying states of anger, sorrow, guilt, and shame that support many states and habits of harm. Likewise you become better able to ease and transform more and more intangible and tangible harm so as to divert more and more resources to processes of healing and cure.

When your transformation is well under way, you can take note of your healing states, habits, and abilities and help them to grow and develop as you change. You can then bring them into your being and becoming and so apply them to your creation of a new and better life. When you are ready, the change that rises in you may overflow into life in time and aid those who are near to you and who are still holding states and habits of harm.

When you transform harmful states and habits, you become like a heroin addict who has joined a loving community that can slake the deep thirst for all forms of love that led to the addiction. Filled with this love, the addict can taper the use of heroin over time and then, when ready, take great joy in being free of the slavery of drug use. The addict then becomes an example to others who desire love and lack faith that they will be able to find it and so cure themselves.

Right Effort. When you take on and transform harmful states and habits, you may tend to make one of two errors, namely, to try too little or to try too hard. In other words, you may tend to slack or to strive. If you try too little, you cannot succeed; if you try too much, you deepen the harm you are trying to ease.

With right effort, you hone your degree of effort with life experience and learn to stay on the razor's edge that divides want from excess. The ancients compared right effort to the tuning of a stringed instrument. If the strings are too slack, the note sounded is absent or muddy; if the strings are too taut, the sound is screechy. Only with the right tension can the strings produce a beautiful sound that you and others can enjoy.

When you develop the healing ability of right effort, which you attune to your present state, you can apply it to all aspects of your sevenfold body and your life. For example, you can increase your fleshly fitness by doing the right amount of physical activity, that is, an amount that enhances your strength without causing setback or injury. When you use right effort you are like a person who chooses a calling, learns with training and experience to practice it with ease, and stays at the cutting edge of the calling to discern and try the new possibilities that are coming into being.

Wisdom. Wisdom is the ability to always transform your awareness, understanding, and perceptions and to apply this transformation easily and effectively and with right effort. That is, it is the ability to use all experience, direct and indirect, to sync with life and time as you discern and realize your deepest purpose. When you are wise, you interpret experience through all seven levels of your body and use all of what you learn to enhance your life and all other sources of life without regard to time or distance.

When we over-rely on any one level of the body, it becomes like an actor who grabs the microphone, stands in the spotlight, and is willing create any drama or distraction that may draw your attention away from all other things, including those that are both urgent and important. For example, if you focus too much on your energy body, it may rivet your understanding to fantastic notions or bewitch you with a desire for power. If you focus too much on your part of interbeing, you may attend to endless urgent pleas that distract you from what is important. If you focus too much on your sensations you may get caught up in a never-ending stream of details that are trivial and also addictive.

With wisdom, you do not focus too heavily on any one level of the body. You do not waste precious opportunities because you are caught up in expanding your awareness, lost in a labyrinth of ideas, or obsessed by one or more habitual responses. With wisdom, you move your focus easily and at will so as to observe concerns and events that relate to being, becoming, and cure.

When you are wise, you have the awareness of an artist who has a new vision and is nurturing and realizing it; the understanding of a theorist who is gelling a new idea; and the perceptions of a mimic, who is also an actor, and can thus mirror someone on sight and then read their states and habits for insights and perspectives. When you are wise, you can integrate your sevenfold body and sync with life in time.

Synchronization with Life in Time

Since before you were conceived, your body has been gaining and gathering experiences as impressions, some of which live on in you today as the living past. Some elements of this past support your healing and cure, as when vivid memories of love sustain you in times of trial. Others may do harm, as when harmful states such as defeat, apathy, or avarice sustain your living past and link it with harmful habits of fear or dislike. These harmful states and habits divide you from the present and prevent you from starting afresh.

When any part of your living past is harming self or others, it is time for you to put it to rest. Doing so will help to sync your body with life in time and to better support your ongoing processes of healing and cure. In other words, putting the past to rest deepens your grounding in life in time. This in turn enables you to find new sources of healing and cure; to respond to the present rather than the past; and to put away idle or harmful notions that conceal the real as well as the ideal. As you put the past to rest, you can better sync with life in time by integrating your sevenfold body, resolving your time debts, and deepening your ties to interbeing.

To integrate the sevenfold body, you can practice bringing your awareness or perceptions to every other level of the body; attend to any level of the body that has received too little notice; or follow a set of practices like that detailed in the *Manual*, in which you join flesh to energy to create vitality and so on until you have joined each level to the next.

To sync with the moving edge of time, you can detect and resolve your time debts. These are burdens that came into you early in life or that you created or took on more recently. Those burdens belong to the living past and can be thought of as personal and shared debts that you can pay and put to rest and so free your sevenfold body to sync with life and time. That is, when you pay or forgive your debts, they cease to hold you back. You can then move freely toward a new and better future.

For example, if you were born into a family that held past trauma, such as memories of a natural disaster, poverty, or war, you may have taken in a set of habits that still define you as a victim or perpetrator. Rather than allow such tenacious perceptions as self-pity, contempt, resentment, or aggression limit your body or your life, you can discern and transform those states and habits of harm. For example, you can work through your memories until they lose their charge and then leave them behind. At the same time, you can join with others in offsetting one or more lasting wrongs.

When you have integrated your sevenfold body, resolved some personal and shared time debts, and deepened your ties with life in time, you can turn your attention to the moving front of life in time and see how to move toward it so as to begin afresh. As you do this, you will open to new and better ways of being in the world.

When you come into sync with life in time you are like a nation that has suffered through a great crisis and that carries great burdens and that has not healed through growth and development. It is now taking stock of old harm and new and trying old and innovative forms of healing and cure. As it takes small steps forward, it begins to learn how to retire processes of harm, to sustain and enhance the web of life, and to envision a better future shared by all life.

Dynamic Equipoise

All of your healing abilities contribute to dynamic equipoise, that is, to the tendency of your processes to continue as they are and, at the same time, to change at their present rate. Your equipoise is like the tendency that an object has when falling toward the earth. You are generally as unaware of your dynamic equipoise as of racing through space with the Earth, which speeds around the sun as it spins on its axis.

With dynamic equipoise, you can start processes of change that continue and that increase at a constant rate. That is, you can seed and guide your healing and cure in sync with life in time, speeding some processes and slowing others as needed. By using intentions as guideposts, you can guide your views, concepts, and habits in keeping with your surroundings and align them so as to create a new and better life that is interwoven with interbeing.

Thus, you can enhance your dynamic equipoise in the context of interbeing by strengthening abilities that enhance your part of interbeing, such as conscience, responsiveness, adaptability, and robustness.

Conscience. In sevenfold healing, conscience is the ability to see what is healing for self and others, to value the strength that comes of that healing, and to act in ways that realize that healing now and forever. With conscience, you can form dynamic principles that support you to enhance, rather than to detract from, your purpose and your present goals. When you form these principles, that is, the ethics that shape your life strategies, you can use them to guide your tangible and intangible actions so as to end old sources of harm and error and to ease new harm as you meet it.

When you hold your conscience with your healing states, and your dynamic principles with healing abilities such as altruism, you can ease and multiply your healing and cure. You can also keep tabs on your principles and heal them as you heal your body and your life and so enable them to better support ongoing healing and cure. For example, as you grow in kind responsibility and gentle prudence, you can open the gateways that limit the free flow of life energy, information, and healing and cure in self and others.

If your healing and cure are like the rope bridge across the chasm of illness, and your intentions are like the destination on the other side, your dynamic principles are like the floor planks that support

74

your feet and like the guiderails that you can grasp with your hands to keep steady in high winds and to avoid a disastrous fall.

Responsiveness. At any given time, your sevenfold body is adjusting your myriads of interrelated processes to suit your conditions. Some of the adjustments happen automatically, as when an airy sigh refreshes your lungs or your ligaments steady a turned ankle. Others happen slowly or with effort, as when your metabolism shifts with the seasons or you learn how to use a new kind of electronic device.

Over time, any abilities or habits that you use in the same way or that you do not use at all become brittle or weak, especially if you are not playful or do not mature. To awaken your abilities and habits, and to engage them in your sevenfold transformation, you can note and enhance your habits and abilities of healing and cure as you go and can adjust them in keeping with your intentions in ways that suit your circumstances.

With responsiveness, you can be described as practical, sensible, coordinated, savvy, nimble, graceful, or adroit. You can monitor and adjust to changing realities so as to continue to further your intentions. When you are responsive, you are like a mule who stays balanced while carrying a shifting rider down the steep and uneven trails that go from the Grand Canyon's rim to the banks of the Colorado River far below.

Adaptability. To paraphrase Shakespeare, the course of true healing never will run smooth. You are bound to meet challenges, setbacks, failures, and barriers, some of which may be expected and trivial and others of which may be shocking and devastating. By expecting bumps in the road, you can prepare to learn from experience and to respond to events in ways that further healing and cure.

You can compare this learning to that of a toddler, that is, you can try and fall and try again until you become able to crawl, to walk, and to run. When you learn from experience, you can observe the world anew and glean from it new insights, joys, and perspectives. You can develop the freedom and mobility to explore the web of life in time and to discern and trace its threads of healing and cure. When your adaptability is strong, you can meet any reality without falling down or staying down. You can cope well with all events, including those that interrupt your life.

When you are adaptable, you are like a temporary worker who is able to go into any setting, to work in it effectively, and to enjoy all that it has to offer while eluding or passing through its perils and staying ready to go on the next job. When you are adaptable in the course of your healing and cure, you can fall in love with life and love it steadfastly for the rest of your days.

Robustness. As you learn to respond to life dynamically and to adapt to it ethically, you can also learn to recover from blips in the course of sevenfold healing and cure. Without robustness, you may be brittle, breakable, or baffled in times of success or failure. With robustness, you can recover with ease and thereby thrive over time.

When your robustness is strong, you avoid lapsing into harmful states or habits or you recover so quickly that little or no harm is done. You will also be able to deepen, broaden, and extend your healing states until you can abide in them easily and constantly through stresses of joy or trials of hardship.

If processes of healing and cure are like a boat, your robustness is like the charts that guide you past shores and shoals, the rope and anchor that hold you steady in times of calm or crisis, and the sextant that reveals your way even when you are tossed by high seas and separated from electricity or satellites.

Chapter 4. Habits for Cure

The habits that prepare you to create self-guided cure are like those that enable you to learn something new. They are informal, that is, based on subjectivity and common sense, and also formal, that is, objective and subject to scrutiny and dialogue. The habits that enable your cure are thus like those that enhance empiricism, that is, the formal processes of learning from experience.

Now, at the end of the modern era, clinical science is reaching the limits of modern methods. Past studies have depended heavily on the aggregation and analysis of data gathered with the assumption that people with the same diagnosis can be grouped together or that they can be divided into groups based on one or more factors. Now that your life has been interrupted by illness or injury, you know from experience that your illness or injury has been unique and so will be the course of your sevenfold healing and cure. You therefore know that there is at least one flaw in the old methods.

You also already know that there is more than one flaw. Because your healing and cure are tangible as well as intangible, and personal as well as shared, you know that the causes and effects of illness are more like a web than like an event or a series of events. You can see this when you look at studies of smoking and disease, which show that smoking can cause many diseases and that those particular diseases can have many causes.

Enjoying healing states and habits is like spending time at a retreat in a luxurious spa or an ancient watering place. Enjoying states and habits of cure is like spending time in a garage laboratory where you try new things so as to envision and to build a new life. That is, you may heal by delving into the intangible and the ineffable; you will find and create cure with the tangible and measurable.

Cure brings understanding to the fore, and includes tasks such as breaking down signs and symptoms, forming them into problems, finding pieces of sevenfold cure, and putting those pieces together to create a complete cure. As you create this cure, you can use your experience as a guide. In other words, you can find your purpose in time and events and use it to guide your ongoing healing as you form a new life that is better than any you can now imagine.

States and Habits for Cure

States and habits of cure enable you to discern, isolate, and dissect away barriers to healing and cure and to pinpoint and put together parts of your sevenfold cure. While healing and cure both rely on understanding, they do so in unlike ways. In healing, you rely on understanding to unify and integrate your sevenfold body; in cure you rely on it to analyze your life, that is, to take your life apart in your mind so that you can put it together in a new and more fulfilling way.

Cure is like the snake venom that Hippocrates of Kos used as a medicine over two millennia ago. In the right dose, it cured his patients. In low doses it did nothing; in high doses it destroyed them. To recognize and mete out doses of cure that are right for you at present, you can rely on your strong processes of healing.

You will know that your healing processes are strong enough to support cure when you have transformed your most burdensome habits of harm, can abide in strong healing states at will, can apply your healing abilities with ease under all circumstances, and can transform new harmful states and habits as they form. Your healing processes will then be strong enough to support and to ensure a smooth, sensible, and effective cure.

The reason to become strong in healing before creating your cure is that while healing and cure both entail processes of destruction, those that enable cure can overwhelm your healing and push you into crisis. For example, if you discover a source of harm outside yourself, your habits of cure may overwhelm your habits of healing, and you may try to attack that source. You may get lost in harmful states of rage or despair and awaken dormant habits of harm such as hate speech or violence. You may then create a needless crisis for yourself and others, and so burn through your healing and cure and that of others and so spread destruction like wildfire.

When you take charge of your cure, and learn to guide it well, you are like a trapeze artist who is performing a hazardous stunt. Your healing processes are like the safety net that frees you to do your best without fear of doing damage to self or others. To ease your way into cure, you can form and enhance habits that strengthen both healing and cure, such as those noted below.

The Check In. With this habit, you can check your sevenfold state of being whenever you feel distracted, confused, or worn down. For example, you can check your energy directly by seeing if it is low grounded and relaxed and indirectly by seeing if your breath is easy and your hips are relaxed.

If your energy body or any other part of your sevenfold body is not in a healing state, you may be able to enhance your ease by taking a big cleansing sigh. If you like, you can sigh loudly enough for others to notice and thus invite them to share your ease. After a moment, you can see if anything is amiss, as when you sense a harmful state of lack or apathy or a harmful habit of anger, sorrow, or greed. If you sense a harmful state or habit, and can pinpoint its causes, you can take timely action to abate those causes. If the cause remains hidden, you can gently invite it to appear to you. If it does not appear, you can allow your perceptions to develop over time until you can see the causes of your harmful state or habit and can find good ways to abate those causes.

Compassionate Reason. With this habit, you combine the synthesis of kind compassion with the analysis and division of sound judgment. By combining these habits to realize your intentions for healing and cure, you can balance them and so avoid relying too much on active acceptance on the one hand and active change on the other.

Unlike passive tolerance, or Freudian introjection or projection, compassionate reason is active, discerning, and embodied. It is intangible and ineffable, and yet you can feel its imprint in your body through the life energy that centers, fills, flows through, and heals your sevenfold body and, through your part of interbeing, the web of life in time.

Compassionate reason entails habits of healing such as love and union as well as habits of cure such as reason and deep dialogue. It thus holds safe harmful states that may accompany reason, such as anger, domination, aggression, or greed, as well as harmful habits of force that range from subtle unconscious manipulation to obvious intentional violence.

To grasp compassionate reason, you can use the Sanskrit mantra "om mani padme hum," which invites the hard, cold diamond of wisdom into the soft, sweet lotus of the heart. Or you can consider Asian traditions that unite the heart and mind rather than divide them in the way of Abelard or Descartes. You can also use a practice of meditation to contemplate the finite and the infinite through the eye of the heart in the way of Jesus and his followers.

Competitive Cooperation. With this habit, you can work through forms of personal and interpersonal discord to unify your sevenfold body, interbeing, and life in time. By contending in dialogue, you can express, hone, and advocate a point of view based on your personal experience, both tangible and intangible. By embracing other points of view, you can integrate your experience with that of others and thus bring together and learn from the lives and thinking of many.

With competitive cooperation, you can use discord to enlarge your worldview until it can take in many points of view that combine to reveal more than you have seen before. And, rather than draw boundaries to define self, friend, and foe, which lead to friction that creates more heat than light, you can discern and transform barriers to concord, such as harmful habits of aggression, secrecy, or pleasing. You can create circumstances in which to use good will to forge accord and thereby to create shared healing and cure.

When you practice deep dialogue, you can learn from indigenous peoples, Quakers, and others who have experience with consensus. You can raise concerns; step up or step back to allow free and equal participation; speak in turn as the spirit moves you; listen deeply to diverse views; respond with kindness, ethics, creativity, and sense; and become able to form and develop an ever-deepening shared awareness with all whom you know.

Embodiment of Change. With this habit, you can recognize that each level, or aspect, of the sevenfold body includes processes of destruction and creation and that you can shift the balance toward creation by healing your harmful states and habits as you envision your cure.

Because this habit supports your inborn dynamism, that is, your inborn capacity for change, and is active, discerning, and embodied,

80

you can use it to sustain the fluidity of your states and habits as you effect healing and cure. You can thus use your sense of relief and wellbeing to discern the changes that are right for you at any given point in time.

When you guide one process of change, you are like a person who is learning to ride a bicycle. You are applying inborn abilities such as balance and strength to learning a skill that others share and that you and they may play with, use, or rely on in the future. When you guide many processes of change, you are like the manager who is guiding the focus and harmony of a troupe of jugglers who toss clubs back and forth as they walk a long distance in sync with each other and with their surroundings.

Fearless Prudence. With this habit, you can open to new possibilities free of harmful states of fear. With fearless prudence, you can let go of harmful habits prompted by states of fear, such as thoughtless, daft, or irresponsible impulses or ingrained habits of avoidance, desperation, or compulsion, any of which could block or reverse your ongoing processes of healing or cure.

With fearlessness, you accept that the future is always unknown, uncertain, and imperfect; that any decision entails risks as well as benefits; and that nature is so complex that any act, however wise and well intended, will lead to some harm as well as to healing. With fearlessness, you free yourself to choose an act, to note its effects, and to make a wiser choice the next time, that is, to become better able to further your intentions for healing and cure with time.

With prudence, you ease your perceptions and understanding so as to discover habits that distort your responses, such as a tendency to seek or to avoid risks; to try out new habits of response and to observe their effects closely; and to use what you learn to form new insights and perspectives that guide your healing and cure.

With fearless prudence, you open nakedly to the now so as to respond to reality with your wits and to do more healing than harm from a subjective or objective view. With fearless prudence, you

81

can be like a figure skater who is free to try a new triple jump with the aid of a harness that prevents reckless or needless harm.

Gracious Disengagement. With this habit, you can be open to others and engage them fully while taking care to support your states and habits of healing and cure. With this habit, you can be grounded in shared interbeing and yet conserve energy, prevent harm, and allow processes of healing and curing to unfold in their own time.

With graciousness, you can spend time with others with ease and enjoy their company as they enjoy yours. With disengagement, you can withdraw from them before overtaxing your resources and thereby weakening your healing states and habits. You can also limit the time you spend with those who cannot create healing states for themselves, who undermine your healing states or habits, or who create and share harmful states and habits that you are not presently able to transform.

With gracious disengagement, you are like a social networker who has the gift of friendship and who has the personal, interpersonal, and interspecies agency to be able to enjoy anyone's company, to bring together those who enjoy each other, and to avoid or to defuse awkward situations.

Patient Insistence. With this habit, you can take time to get to know your problems, to identify possible solutions, and to use trial and error to put together solutions that take you closer to becoming healing and realizing cure. As you pursue those solutions, you can stick to them and adjust them as needed until you are creating and sustaining a new and better life.

With patience, you can avoid wasting resources on problems that have yet to show known patterns or on solutions that are as yet unknown or unavailable. You can recognize that as in comedy, timing is everything in healing and cure, and that your solution will work best if you wait until your problem is ripe for it.

With insistence, you can discern barriers that impede your healing and cure and decide whether to transform them into opportunities or to hold fast and to pass through them. With insistence, you will be able to do what is right for as long as you need to do it at those times when you have chosen to endure an obstacle to healing and cure rather than to transform it.

With patient insistence, you do not rush or take desperate shortcuts that may divert you from your goal, nor do you take no for an answer. Rather than alter your practices or processes of healing or cure, you take whatever respites you need and go the distance to reach your goals.

With patient insistence, you are like a person who has nothing to lose and who starts a business, learns the nitty-gritty tasks that make it work, and then picks it up by the bootstraps and carries it to success. That is, you are taking on a new and daring venture with the expectation that success may be long in coming, will come in its own time, and will offer up some obstacles that call for endurance and tenacity rather than for change.

Persistent Ingenuity. With this habit, you keep to your intentions for healing and cure while engaging your ongoing experience with abilities like curiosity and creativity, which can turn up new and better solutions for your problems. Persistent ingenuity enables you to discover pieces of your cure and bring them into your life even as you continue to hone your ingenuity. With persistent ingenuity, you look to your experience to find new ways of solving your life problems and keep trying them as you make your way to cure.

With persistent ingenuity, you can become like a student of music who follows the teaching method developed by Shinichi Suzuki. That is, you gently challenge your abilities and then learn in your own way and in your own time by relying on and enhancing your present abilities and by allowing those to bring to the fore others that have been weak, hidden, dormant, or complex. Thus, by using and enjoying the abilities that you have now, you can note and develop others and thereby reach your full flowering.

If you have, for many years, worked at a single role in a complex system, you may have lost touch with your creativity and have let others take charge. You may have become like the last person on an assembly line, who struggles to keep up with decisions made by the engineers and workers who have come before you. If so, you can revive your persistent ingenuity by trying to discern, develop, and adopt new pieces of cure and by responding to any and all failures with new efforts.

With persistent ingenuity, you become like an intrepid explorer who is undaunted by icy peaks or valleys of shadows and who remains ever confident of blazing a path over the horizon to a better life.

Personalization of Generalities. Now, at the end of the modern era, chances are good that you have access to more information than you can put to use. That is, you, like radar readers, radiologists, and forecasters, may be looking for rare signals in a sea of noise. To detect signals that may be of use, you can look at the experiences of others and apply them to your own, that is, you can try to personalize generalities.

With generalities, you identify signals that arise from groups. These signals are often easier to find and to measure than those that may arise from any one person. You can thus learn more, and can do so more rapidly and completely, by learning from interbeing as you learn from your part of interbeing. That is, you can ease your way ahead by taking both into account as you devise pieces of cure.

With personalization, you can take into account the fact that we are not all alike and that your healing and cure will be as unique as your life experience. You can then examine possibilities that you glean from personal and shared experience and can try on various pieces of cure and use those that work for you.

You can also weigh your risks and benefits. That is, you can be like a scientist who finds that aluminum increases the risk of dementia and who continues to use antiperspirants with aluminum. That is, you can see the risks to a large population and then, if it suits you and your circumstances, can choose to accept a certain risk to gain a particular benefit.

When you personalize generalities, you are like a person who gets a companion dog based on the breed and who then, after coming to know the dog, sees that the dog is an individual unlike any other.

Prepared Forgiveness. When you anticipate that unfolding life is an admixture of what time will reveal to be life and death, healing and harm, and truth and error and that our intelligence can wonder at the ongoing exploration of genesis and contribute actively to the ongoing adjustments that reduce death, harm, and error, you can remain ready to see self and others as they are and to proactively participate in the spontaneous realization of life, healing, and truth. In other words, you can anticipate and recognize the archetypal truth personified in Shiva, that is, that creation entails ongoing destruction. When you see this, you can gently and kindly nurture the life that is always arising even as you ease decay away with care. You can open radically to reality without inviting or accepting harm and without forming unrealistic expectations that can leave you fearful, angry, let down, or abandoned. Instead, you can meet harm with forgiveness that diminishes it with awareness, compassion, altruism, prudence, and proactive change.

With prepared forgiveness, you have the chance to respond well in any circumstance, which will in turn enable you to open to more phenomena, including those that may have prompted upset in the past. It also enables ready transformation of unwelcome actions. With prepared forgiveness you can more quickly and easily develop equanimity and other healing abilities as well and thereby do less and less harm and effect greater and greater healing and cure.

With prepared forgiveness, you are like a diplomat who can read people well, accept them as they are, and converse easily and effectively with friends and enemies alike. You expect nothing in particular, forego free punishment of self or others, and pay heed to interbeing. With prepared forgiveness, you can engage the good in self and others as you leave or transform the rest.

Proactive Responsiveness. With proactive responsiveness, you can meet any event actively and consciously and thus can respond to what is new in the moment rather than to the past that formed your habits.

When you are proactive, you do not wait for healing and cure to come to you; you seek them out. You enhance your awareness and understanding with curiosity, glean new insights and perspectives with experience, and, when you discern a possible source of cure, go after it, learn what you can about it, and prudently try it.

When you are responsive, you are ready to make the most and the best of any and all chances for healing or cure that you meet by intent or by chance. You remain open to new possibilities so as to playfully explore any that you encounter. When you find a potential cure, you can learn more about it, try it out and, if suitable, bring it into the new life that you are creating.

Being proactive and responsive is like shaking hands with the universe; you extend your hand in invitation, wait prudently and fearlessly for any hand proffered in return, and use all of your sevenfold body to gauge your grasp and your new connection.

Sacred Irreverence. With this habit, you can sustain an appreciation of the miraculous nature of all phenomena without giving up authority or responsibility for your body or your life. That is, you can freely express wonder and gratitude free of bonds such as uniformity or conformity. You can marvel at life and remain open to its grace and yet question it and probe it deeply enough to reveal more and more that has been hidden and now is new. In other words, you can regard the heavens with your feet firmly grounded on the earth.

With awareness of the sacred, you can abide in healing states of wonder and joy, extend your interbeing far into the web of life and time, and experience the limitless compassion of the infinite free of tangible or intangible barriers. You can sustain a big-hearted view of life in time that nurtures the opening of your flawed and finite understanding, which will always be provisional, incomplete, and slow to respond to the dynamic nature of life.

With irreverence, you can question anything and everything, that is, kindly pose no-holds-barred questions that may reveal the nature and meaning of things old and new. You can challenge or beguile the gateways of your sevenfold body to open to the full spectrum of reality, and so take the chance to see what you have not seen before. You can apprehend your problems more clearly and fully and comprehend them in ways that enable you build a better life.

With sacred irreverence, you can be like an inspector who feels no qualms about going into the basement of the temple of your mind to seek out signs of rot, termites, and rats so as to remake it free of hidden sources of harm.

Selective Participation. With selective participation, you can engage fully, consciously, and carefully with interbeing. That is, you can note the practices and processes that will further your healing and cure and engage them as you transform or leave the rest. That is, you can conserve your resources and also deepen your grounding.

With selectiveness, you can divert resources such as awareness and attention from harm to healing and cure. With participation, you enhance your grounding and sync and synergize with life in time. In other words, you use your resources wisely to realize healing and cure, and so avoid needless stresses and setbacks. As you advance in healing change, you can become less selective and participate more fully knowing that you can make use of any experience to strengthen and extend your healing and cure.

With selective participation, you are like a voyageur who is floating downstream in a canoe, who portages around rapids and falls while learning to steer with the current and to negotiate higher and faster rapids, and who can then easily navigate the rest of the way.

Stepwise Sequencing. With this habit, you sort out your priorities every time things change, as when you reach a new stage of healing or you change jobs or move house.

With a stepwise approach, you can periodically take stock of your life and decide whether your present processes of healing and cure are making the best use of your resources. If not, you can think of how best to use your resources to further your intentions.

With sequencing, you form a working strategy by which to match your resources to your goals. As you progress, and your dynamic sevenfold body shifts, and life in time changes around you, you can form a new strategy that suits your present circumstances. That is, you can take the next step by reviewing your priorities and deciding how to pursue them.

With stepwise sequencing, you revise your priorities so that you focus on those that do the most for you in the moment and over time. That is, you peg your priorities to your present reality and adjust your strategies as needed.

With stepwise sequencing, you are like a coach who is choosing team members to play in a game. You bring some of them in to develop their skills and to see what they can do. You can then play the ones who help the team and bench those who do not. Over time, you can also retire some players and recruit new ones.

Skeptical Trust. With this habit, you can sustain appropriate doubt as you discern the practices and processes of healing and cure that you can rely on at present. That is, you question your ongoing decisions and use your doubt to deepen your basic trust in your life and in your growing ability to learn from it.

With trust, you can rest your confidence in your unique unfolding story and so respond with relative ease to those setbacks that are bound to arise through confusion, error, or mischance. That is, you can trust your dynamic sevenfold body to respond to experience and trust your response to reveal what you need to learn in order to move ahead as you realize healing and cure.

With skepticism, you can recognize and accept the unknown and respond to it proactively and rationally, that is, with awareness and wits rather than with harmful habits such as dislikes that prompt anger, avoidance, hatred, or cravings, which can prompt glutting, bingeing, or addiction.

With skeptical trust, you can try any tool devised by a scientist or mystic and see if it opens your body to the full spectrum of the unknown and unseen and ensure that this opening does not lead to excessive credulity, flights of fancy, or other habits that reflect weak or absent grounding in life in time. Put differently, you can explore the unknown and unseen without losing your grip.

With skeptical trust you become like a monk who is following in the footsteps of Saint Francis of Assisi, or like a scientist who is extending the theories of Einstein. You see in the natural world what others do not and enable those who come after you to keep faith with the hidden order of the universe as they steadily discern more of the miraculous and infinite unknown.

Strategic Nonparticipation. With strategic nonparticipation, you can bypass avenues of healing and cure that are unlikely to do you any good, as with responses that do not match your problems, that do not support your unique healing or cure, that put motion before action, or that apply red tape to your dynamic sevenfold body.

With strategy, you can weigh possible responses to your problems, try those that may enhance your healing or cure, and sustain any that do so. With nonparticipation, you can refuse any care that does not suit your healing or cure, as with treatments that heal or cure others but that harm you. With strategic nonparticipation, you can make decisions that are right for you even when they might not be right for others.

With strategic nonparticipation, you are like a bridge player who is holding a poor hand and who decides to pass on a bid. That is, you can look over the resources offered to you, recognize when none is worthy of time or effort, and let others know your opinion.

Timely Triage. With timely triage, you recognize when a problem is serious and give it immediate attention. You avoid common errors such as ignoring urgent problems or overreacting to passing ones. You remain aware of your body's signals and read them wisely so as to respond in the right way at the right time.

With timeliness, you can recognize new or worsening signs of harm as they arise. With triage, you decide whether, when, and how to respond to those signs. With timely triage, you use your experience to hone habits of strong judgment, kind compassion, and effective action by which you can respond promptly and wisely to your dynamic sevenfold body and can consult others as needed.

With timely triage, you become like a medic who can make tough decisions on the spot under pressure. That is, you can see what is important, assess it objectively, and respond well in the moment.

Analysis of Signs and Symptoms

When your life was interrupted by illness or injury, your signs may have led your consultants to make a definite diagnosis with a simple prognosis and a clear course of treatment that you readily accepted. Or, you may have experienced signs and symptoms that failed to fit a familiar pattern or fell outside your system of care; if so, you may face the task of defining your problems, detecting their causes, and creating a cure from scratch. You may be obliged to become a medical detective like those in the stories of Berton Roueché.

To become your own detective, you can keep a list of your signs and symptoms, that is, your tangible and intangible difficulties; identify patterns based on timing, prompts, and effects; group your difficulties into problems; and look for clues as to their causes and cures in things that make them worse or better.

For example, your difficulties may include sour stomach, bloating, cough, pain and tingling in the legs, face rash, fluey feelings, and irregularity. As you observe these difficulties, you may see that the sour stomach and rash occur together; that the cough and nerve pain are both prompted by swampy areas or "sick" buildings; and that the fluey feelings and irregularity are relieved by an elimination diet. You can then organize your list into three problems. Later, if you note that the first group is related to the last, you can organize your list into two problems. As you track these problems, you may find that certain foods prompts or eases all of your symptoms and that you have only one problem. Eventually, you sort out your problems and form a regimen that eases all of them.

As you do this detective work, you are like a sleepy woolworker who is sorting balls of colored yarn in the pre-dawn darkness. At first you may try to sort them by size or feel. Then, as you awaken and "clear the cobwebs," and your black and white night vision gives way to color vision, you become able to see and sort your balls of yarn by color so that you can use them to weave the pattern of your new life.

As you pinpoint your problems, and seek out pieces of cure, you can consult with others who may have heard of problems like yours and have found ways to ease them. You can begin by consulting doctors of mainstream medicine who have access to modern gains. If they cannot help you, your counselors and bodyworkers may be able to help you. If not, you can consult other experts and network with people who are in similar straights.

By sustaining your healing states and habits as you hone your states and habits of cure, including processes of analysis, you can avoid harmful states such as sorrow, fear, or apathy and harmful habits such as blame or despair. With strong healing states and habits, you can wield the sharp tools of analysis without harming self or others.

Step-by-Step Cure—Taking the First Step

When you have defined your problems, and have identified those things that prompt or ease them, you are ready to take the step of gathering components, or pieces, of your cure. In the late modern era, cure has been defined as the end of fleshly disease; in sevenfold healing it is defined the creation of a new and better life. With this definition, your cure will be ongoing and inclusive, and you will be able to center it in your body rather than in your systems of care and thereby take charge of it. You will also be able to support your relief, wellbeing, and healing change as you create your new life.

When you view your cure as stepwise, you can solve one problem at a time, and so bring along your process of analysis. That is, you can eliminate some problems and simplify those that remain. You can also proceed through prudent trial and error rather than waiting for the slow wheels of modern science to turn, which may or may not happen in your lifetime.

Likewise, this definition enables you to address intangible and unknown sources of illness that scientists and doctors may feel obliged to ignore but that you cannot. You can thus continue healing as you take tangible steps to change your body and your life.

When you use this definition, you can heal with life in time and still consult with doctors who can access to the best care that the late modern era has to offer.

When you consult with your doctor, and you hold the view that cure consists of creating a new and better life, you can take note of and pass over any late modern ideas that may be working against you. You can take note of and decline unnecessary limits to healing or cure imposed by fields such as law, economics, religion, science, engineering, or management and that prevent you and your doctor from learning from life. You can note and decline treatments that do you more harm than good, as may be so with any treatment, and is likely when systems of care are so complex and centralized as to be oblivious of and unresponsive to your sevenfold body. You can also focus on your life rather than on ailments that may or may not be valid and that may not support your healing or cure.

As with the analysis of signs and symptoms noted in the previous section, you can use the sevenfold definition of cure to form and hone habits by which to find, ease, and end processes that are causing pain and suffering. As you do this, you can prudently try various cures and allow your life experience to be your guide in choosing and using the cures that are best for you at present.

When you have seen and defined a problem, and have pinpointed one or more things that prompt it, you can try to ease or end the problem by avoiding the prompts. For example, if you find that some foods or alcoholic beverages cause pain and tingling in your legs, inability to find words, or problems with position or balance, you can realize cure by removing those foods or beverages from your diet. That is, you can use what you learn to ease your suffering and to bring a cure into your new and better life.

As you proceed, you may note that your cures bear a complex relationship to illnesses or injury and to their causes and effects. At the start, you may expect one cure to end your pain and suffering, and it may do so, but you may also find that the more cures you bring into your new life, the better it will be.

One reason for this is that illness or injury and healing or cure will have complex effects, and those effects may unfold for days or for decades and may each impact the other. This complexity can baffle you and thus present a challenge. If you get lost in the complexity you will make errors of confusion; if you simplify the complexity too early or in the wrong way you will make mistakes of ignorance. To find the simplicity that will yield your cure, you may have to bide your time and act when ready. Defining cure as creating a better life gives you the time you need to do this.

As you look for the simplicity that enables action, you can think of each cause of each problem as resulting from a "causal pie" or from a web of "multiple hits." A causal pie is like a perfect storm; it happens when many factors come together. A causal pie may seem to have only one piece if that piece is the limiting factor, that is, if it is missing and adding it completes a causal pie that is already in place. A web of multiple hits becomes more fixed as it leads to more tangible effects. By seeking out causes and cures that are well "upstream," you can find those causes that are easiest to alter.

As you penetrate the complex and the uncertain, you can rely on the healing ability of right effort, which will save you from the impatience that might cause you to jump to conclusions and also from the delay that could lead you to hold out for impossible clarity. You can apply right effort by relying on your states and habits of healing as you gently probe your experience and use your states and habits of cure to try new things, note the effect, and to become cure as you become healing.

You can gauge the progress of your healing and cure by checking in with your body's central channel and your grounding in interbeing. You can also note the strength of your healing states and enjoy any times when you become so rich in life energy that it brims over into your part of interbeing. You can also note any growing resilience to colds, seasonal allergies, stress, and other passing sources of unease or illness. When you detect signs of greater resilience and of greater relief, wellbeing, and healing change, you will know that you are growing closer to realizing your ultimate intentions.

As you become cure, curiosity will lead you to new discoveries and to new ways of making discoveries. At the same time, creativity will engage your spirit of play and lead you to delight in creating cures that become part of your new second nature, which is already coming into being inside your sevenfold body. As you create your new and better life, you will be like the prince who undertakes a quest by traveling long distances, cutting through dense hedges, and scaling high walls so as to discover, awaken, and embrace the beauty that is sleeping within.

Step-By-Step Cure—Taking Further Steps

As you bring cures into your new and better life, you go through important rites of passage. To make sense of them, you can think of yourself as like an autobiographer who is rewriting your story. To enhance this process, you can use the exercises below to mark the end of the old life and the creation of the new one.

Rite of Passage Ritual. One ritual by which to enact change is to write your problems on a slip of paper and to burn it. For example, at the end of a week, month, or year of healing and cure, you can set aside an hour or more in which to discern what is sacred to you now; what problems you have eased or ended since you began to heal (or since your last ritual); and what cures you are bringing into your new life now. You can then write your problems on one slip of paper and your cures on another.

You now design and carry out a ritual that suits you. For example, you can put the slip of paper with your cures in a safe place such as in the pocket of a bag that you always carry or in a drawer by your bedside. That way you can look at it whenever you like.

You can then make your progress tangible by safely burning the slip of paper on which you wrote your problems. For instance, you can place a votive candle in a holder and place the holder on a fire-resistant surface. Then you can make the ritual your own by reading a few words of poetry, wearing a special item, visualizing the fire as a sacrifice, saying a favorite prayer, or doing something else that engages you in a meaningful rite of passage.

Now, take the slip of paper on which you wrote your problems and fold it or roll it into a scroll. Finally, light the candle, invoke the sacred, light the scroll and allow it to burn, and then let it drop onto the surface where it can safely burn itself out. Take time to appreciate the progress that you have made and the new life that you are creating.

If it feels right to you, give thanks or offer blessings that express your gratitude for your old life and for what you are doing now to create a better one. If you like this ritual, repeat it when you have eased or ended any problem and are ready to observe another rite of passage. If you don't like this ritual, devise one that suits you.

Stream of Dreams. Prepare for this exercise by setting aside an hour or more in which to write without unwanted interruptions; a place where you can write; and whatever writing materials best support you in the free expression of creative narratives or ongoing trains of thought. If you have trouble finding a good time to write, try a time when others are asleep.

When you sit down to write, set your intentions to describe the most desirable life that you can imagine living in the near future. Before you begin writing, check your state of being. If you are not in a strong healing state, adjust your posture; take a few long, slow deep cleansing breaths; relax your hips; and bring your attention to your crown to deepen your grounding in interbeing and then down to your sacrum to deepen your grounding in the earth.

Now, start writing your story as stream of consciousness, that is, as a flow of ideas free of pauses, second thoughts, or revisions. Allow your thoughts to flow without stopping and sync your writing to the flow of your thoughts. If able, start your story at a point before your life was interrupted and continue through the interruption and the present time into the near future that you are envisioning now as you begin to create your new life.

As you do this, take care to sustain your healing state and to refresh it as needed. Allow your thoughts to form the thread of your story. If you have a new idea and your thoughts form another thread, continue writing the story by following that thread forward. If you lose the thread, gently return to it and continue forward. Write without stopping until your time is up or you finish, whichever comes first.

When you finish, take a moment to note and enjoy any new insights or perspectives that came to you as you were writing. Take another moment to take joy in the new and better life that you are already envisioning and creating. If you like, devote one or more daily formal healing practices to visualizing your new and better life and the means by which you will realize it, including leaving behind your problems and bringing in new cures. Likewise, you can set aside half a day or more for a mini-retreat in which you update your goals and strategies to align with your developing vision.

If you lose your healing state at any time, as when your thoughts veer from inspiring to harrowing, gently refresh your healing state and your grounding. If you are unable to do this, stop the exercise, do what you need to do to recover your healing state, and make a note of your difficulty. You may have run into a part of the living past that is holding you back and that you are not ready to write out. If so, take this as a chance to see if it is time to put that part of your past to rest on your own or with the aid of a trusted friend, wise elder, or consultant.

Alternatively, if you find that you are writing nonsense, that is, that your writing does not reflect your deepest truth, you may be trying to avoid an aspect of the present that you do not want to face or that you are not yet ready to face. If need be, challenge yourself to go deeper, and take whatever time you need to work through your difficulty. Do not use force; allow your strong intentions to guide you to do things that you are ready to do.

You will know that the exercise is working for you when the story that you write freely from your depths is the one that you want to embody and that you are already becoming. When it is working for you, you can return to it whenever you like, as when your body or your circumstances change and you are ready to adapt to them or to change with them.

Memoir. In this exercise, you write a brief story of your life and rewrite it on a regular basis. Depending on how much you like to write, and how well writing helps you to think things through, you may wish to write a few pages, fifty pages, or more. You begin by dividing your life into short chapters based on five- or ten-year time periods, including a five or ten-year period in the future, and start with the chapter that you are most ready to write. As you write each chapter, develop the themes of destruction and creation, that is, discern and describe threads of harm and healing that run through that time in your life. Add a speculative account of your near future in which you extend those threads according to the vision that you have of your new life.

If the living past is troubling you and making it difficult for you to write a chapter or version of your memoir, as when the interruption in your life was so traumatic that you cannot yet revisit it without losing your healing state, you can delay writing that chapter or you can write it as a myth or allegory. Feel free to use your well-grounded imagination as you do this.

For a while, your story may change every year or every day. For example, when your life begins to gel and your healing states grow expansive and resilient, you can ground your story in the key details of your past and present and can extend your story into the future with playful confidence.

Consultation with Doctors and Habitat Restorers

When it comes to restoring the tangible aspects of your flesh and your part of interbeing, chances are good that you will wish to gain the benefit of tangible expertise that you do not possess. This may be simple if you have had good experiences with modern medicine, science, and activism and are ready to apply the gifts of modernity to your tangible healing and cure. This may be complex if you have had bad experiences and are not yet prepared to bring forward the best of our recent shared past.

If you like, you can prepare to make the most of modern gifts by taking stock of the inventions and innovations that transformed healing and cure around the globe. You can give thanks that our forebears used the tools of science and social change to extend the health and happiness of countless lives. You can appreciate that doctors and their partners reduced maternal and infant mortality; devised effective treatments for infections, trauma, and tumors; sparked the hygiene movement that spread clean drinking water and sewage treatment; and developed rapid responses to natural disasters, mass trauma, and epidemics. We can honor our ancestors for transforming many fatal and lasting illnesses or injuries into passing ones and eliminating the ancient scourge of smallpox.

You can also prepare to make the most of modernity by beginning to see and to remedy its shadow side. In other words, you can face the hitherto hidden costs and limitations of modernity and learn to live in a way that resolves any harm that you have done knowingly or unknowingly. It is this new way of living that will heal and cure your time debts and enhance life in time.

Whether or not your relation to modern medicine is simple or complex, the fact that your life was interrupted now at the end of the modern era means that your healing and cure will arise as you come to terms with whatever limits of modernity you may embody. You may have lost your grounding in interbeing by idolizing science and technology on the one hand, or by reacting to it on the other. Or, you may have lost your grounding in interbeing by avoiding responsibility for life in time on the one hand or by taking too much responsibility for it on the other.

If you have lost your grounding in interbeing, you can turn to those that have remained well grounded and who comprehend tangible healing and cure of flesh and interbeing. To seek and make good use of their advice, you may have to mature in ways that are not presently popular. You may be obliged to give up illusions of control, to come to terms with sickness and mortality, and to learn from life rather than from the Internet.

When you are ready to engage modern medicine and, at the same time, to accept its limits, you can seek the advice of your doctor, reconcile that advice with what you know from your sevenfold body and your life, and create a plan that you can use until you are ready to revise it through experience.

You can do the same as you take part in healing and curing your part of interbeing, including the tangible habitat or ecosystem or bioregion to which you belong. You may be able to heal and cure your part of interbeing on your own by engaging in permaculture, tending an Audubon garden, or adopting a forest or field. Or you can join with a group that includes others who have trained as ecologists, zoologists, botanists, or entomologists, or who otherwise have experience that can support you and others to wisely preserve or restore your habitat.

Given the great store of knowledge and noise accumulated in the era of modernity, is likely that you will wish to partner with qualified professionals in healing the tangible parts of flesh and interbeing. To paraphrase Theodore Roosevelt, you will be able to join with them in order to best do what you can, where you are, with what you have and to create and share healing and cure with others who choose to do the same.

Afterword

Sevenfold Healing SYSTEMS*MEDIA*GUILDS is a vision dedicated to those who wish to explore and expand the frontiers of self-guided healing and cure. This vision includes systems and media for chronic illness, as presented in the upcoming second edition of *The Chronic Illness Owner's Manual*; systems and media for fertility and interbeing that are in development; and the formation of Guilds of Founders, Masters, and Guides of Sevenfold Healing and Cure.

To receive periodic updates on Sevenfold Healing, and to follow my story of curing chronic fatigue syndrome, you can use your Internet browser to navigate to 7foldHealing.com or sevenfoldcure.com and to sign up for updates.

Best wishes for your speedy healing and cure,

Beth Alderman, MD MPH, Seattle 2013

Acknowledgment

Thank you for medical and public health education and training to the University of Chicago, Michael Reese Hospital, and the University of Washington; for training to my many Jewish and African American mentors at Michael Reese Hospital and to Professors Pierce Gardner, Monte Lloyd, Richard Mintel, Irwin Rosenberg, Margaret Telfer, Karl Joachim Weintraub, and Noel Weiss and to Joel Mason, Kathryn Miles, Howard Nagatani, Daniel Shuh, Jill Stein, and Hugh Taylor; for mentorship and collegiality in public health practice and research to Drs. Anna Barón, Edward Boyko, Jose Cordero, Janet Daling, Irvin Emanuel, Allan Lock, Ellen Mangione, Lorna Moore, Lorene Nelson, Andy Olshan, Mim Orleans, John Reif, David Savitz, and to many others too numerous to mention; for creativity to those who responded to AIDS by engaging and transforming the world; and for personal advice to Drs. Tracy Johansson, Martin Ross, and Fernando Vega.

Thank you for inspiration and instruction to Granny Gustafson, Grandma Johnson, Aunt Louise, and Uncle Ernie; to my mother and father; to Sherman Alexie Silversong Belcourt, Cynthia Bourgeault, Geshe Doga, Matthew Fox, Tim Harris, Phil Gerson, Geshe Kelsang Gyatso, Derek Hoshiko, Gen Khedrub, Jack Kornfield, Phil Lane Jr., Cara Marianna, Weldon Nisly, Craig Rennebohm, Dezhung Rinpoche, Reggie and Caroline Ray, Sharon Salzberg, Gene Tagaban, and Rebbe Zalman; and to Campion Centre for Ignatian Spirituality, La Casa de Maria, Center for Ethical Leadership, Center for Spiritual Living Seattle, Christian Peacemaker Teams, Compassionate Action Network, The Interfaith Amigos, Miraval Spa, Monkfish Abbey, Nalanda West, Paths to Awakening, St. Stephen's Episcopal Church, Sakya Monastery, SCALLOPS, Seattle Insight Meditation Society, Spiritual Paths Institute, and the Tara Institute.

Thank you for formative dialogue to Dr. Edward Boyko, Will Blades, Rev. Cynthia Bradley, Rabbi Ted Falcon, Marjon Flores,

Phil Gerson, Imam Jamal Rahman, John Malcomson, Timothy Malone, Dr. Lora-Ellen McKinney, Oceanna, and Jane Shofer; thank you for prose instruction and assistance to writing mavens Wendy Call, Andrea Goldsmith, Stephanie Holt, Kathy Kizilos, Jill Kelley, and Eva Silverfine and to the groups that support writing at Hugo House and Victorian Writers' Centre.

And thank you for vision and inspiration to Tony Kushner for sharing the angels; to Drs. María Alvárez Belón and James Orbinski for courage; to The Dalai Lama, the Transcendentalists, Silversong Belcourt, Alice Walker, and Richard Wright for speaking with the voice of love; to Buckminster Fuller, the Living Building Institute, Mike Reynolds, and Frank Lloyd Wright for building better shelter; and to Nancy Wertheimer and Drs. Thomas Chalmers, Paul Farmer, and Tom Hornbein for showing that one mind can matter when it observes life carefully in the belief that what is passing is showing us the way forward.

Glossary

Becoming. In sevenfold healing, becoming is the overall change in your states of being over time. You can become healing and cure by doing practices that enhance your related abilities and habits and that deepen, broaden, and extend your relevant states over time.

Being. In sevenfold healing, being is your inner, subjective state at a given point in time. Your state of being may be healing when you embody relief, wellbeing, and transformation. Your state of being may be curative when you are in a healing state and are taking steps to create a new and better life.

Body (see Sevenfold Body)

Bodyworker. In sevenfold healing, a bodyworker is a consultant who can directly transmit healing states of being or induce them without the aid of drugs or devices through the laying on of hands or the transmission of life energy. Examples of bodyworkers include practitioners of massage, physical therapy, acupuncture, accutonics, healing touch, reiki, Rubenfeld Synergy Work, or healing prayer. Self-guided healers can also learn self-administered forms of bodywork such as yoga, meditation, qi gong, Feldenkreis, or tantra.

Central Channel. Known in Sanskrit as the shushumna nadi, the central channel is the intangible backbone of the energy body that runs from the crown to the pelvis along the front of the spine. This channel forms the core of the energy body, which comprises the dynamic electrical potentials and magnetic fields of the body's matter, especially those created by the nervous tissues, the cardiac conduction system, and the ions that circulate with the body's fluids. The main intangible centers, or chakras, of the energy body are located in this channel.

Chakras. The chakras are the intangible energy centers that relate to the nerve plexi that parallel the spinal cord. Major centers include the crown, brow, throat, heart, epigastric, navel, and sacral chakras. When you center the energy body strongly in the central channel, and balance the energy in the major chakras, you may be able to strengthen the energy body enough to bypass limitations created by damage to electrically active tissues.

Counselor. In sevenfold healing, a counselor is a consultant who is able to aid self-guided healers in removing obstacles to being and becoming healing. An example of such an obstacle is a perceptual barrier linked to harmful states and habits, such as a persecution complex that entails the ongoing giving and receiving of harm. A promising counselor for self-guided healers may be an experienced therapist with training in divinity as well as psychology or in a form of body-oriented psychotherapy such as Rubenfeld Synergy.

Cure. Sevenfold cure is the ongoing creation of a new life that realizes your deepest purpose and that is always becoming better than you could have imagined in the past. This new and better life includes outward, objective changes that have tangible as well as intangible effects.

Dynamic. In sevenfold healing and cure, you recognize that ignoring time adds to harm and that becoming aware of time and working well with it leads to healing and cure. As you pay heed to time, you become aware that everything is dynamic and open to healing and cure and that healing and cure are dynamic and ongoing.

Insight. To heal and cure the intangible aspects of your body, you can observe and assess them and thus become aware of them. You can work from the inside out, as by using insight meditation and the third eye, or from the outside in, as by using journaling or role-playing. In sevenfold healing, you can conceive of this process as bringing your awareness into your understanding and perceptions or as part of integrating your sevenfold body.

Intangible. Not comprised of matter or not measured as matter by modern methods and tools.

Integration. Analyzing the body through the sevenfold model entails focusing on practices and processes that heal and cure each level of the body. Integration opens those processes to all levels of the body and balances them in ways that hinder processes of harm and ease processes of healing and cure. Integration is thus the synthesis that follows sevenfold analysis and transformation.

Intentions. In Sevenfold Healing Systems, you take healing and cure as your ultimate intentions, or goals, and allow those intentions to motivate you and to guide you toward ever greater healing and cure.

Interbeing. Interbeing is the one shared life that includes all seemingly separate sources of generative life. Buddhist monk Thich Nhat Hanh describes interbeing as an ocean of life on which each being appears superficially as a wave. In Progoff Work, interbeing is seen as a deep underground stream; in tantra it is seen as Indra's net.

In sevenfold healing, you can conceive of your part of interbeing as the tangible and intangible connections that join your body with your surroundings. You can then conceive of shared interbeing as all sources of generative life that have ever existed and will ever exist, their dynamic interconnections, and the context of space and time with which interbeing is unfolding. The interconnections include tangible ones, like chemical processes and the birth of descendants, and intangible ones, like personal habits and propagated memories.

Life in Time (see Web of Life)

Perspective. To heal and cure the tangible aspects of your flesh and interbeing, you can observe and assess them indirectly and objectively from the vantage point of interbeing. You can do this from the center by seeing the big picture around you, or from the periphery by seeing your body as a small and distant element of the vast and dynamic expanse of life in time. To develop perspective on your sevenfold body, you can visualize yourself trading places with other people and seeing each level of your body through their eyes.

Practices of Cure. Formal or informal exercises that you use to effect stepwise, tangible changes in your life so that it that is always becoming better than any you could have imagined and is always bringing you closer to fulfilling your deepest dynamic purpose.

Practices of Healing. Formal or informal exercises that you use to initiate, sustain, and enhance processes of transformation that may transpire on any or all levels of the sevenfold body. These processes can be subjective or objective; may yield intangible or tangible results; and will sooner or later transform your body and your life.

Processes of Cure. Dynamic actions that free your sevenfold body of obstacles, yield tangible changes that you can measure indirectly and objectively, or create a new and better life.

Processes of Healing. Dynamic actions that you guide directly and subjectively with the aid of your intentions and that initiate, sustain, or increase your sevenfold relief, wellbeing, and transformation.

Right Effort. In realizing intentions for healing and cure, right effort is midway between slacking and striving; it is therefore the degree of effort that is just right for forming and sustaining progress. Right effort therefore does not err by lapsing, as with apathy, or by leading to fruitless shortcuts, as with desperation.

Sacrum. The sacrum is the bone at the bottom of the lumbar spine that holds the pelvic wings and tailbone.

Scale. In sevenfold healing and cure, you can conceive of scale as comprising three levels, namely, infinitesimal, human, or infinite. The infinitesimal scale includes material objects that are too small to assess through the five senses. The human scale includes material objects that you can assess through the five senses and that form the basis of common sense. The infinite scale includes phenomena that are too big or too universal to assess through the five senses.

Sevenfold Body. In sevenfold healing and cure, the body is conceived of as including seven levels: awareness, understanding, perceptions, sensations, energy, flesh, and interbeing.

Sevenfold Cure. Ongoing, self-guided, intentional, practice-driven, step-by-step creation of a new and better life (see *Practices of Cure.*)

Sevenfold Healing. Ongoing, self-guided, intentional practice-driven, continuous realization of increasing relief, wellbeing, and healing change (see *Practices of Healing.*)

States of Cure. States of being in which you abide in a healing state as you create objective improvement via processes of cure such as analysis, which may at first prompt harmful states like anger.

States of Healing. States of being that you embody to realize ever-greater subjective relief, wellbeing, and healing change.

Tangible. Comprised of matter and measured as matter by modern methods and tools of science.

Time Debts. In sevenfold healing and cure, you conceive of your living, harmful past as consisting of time debts that you can resolve by paying or forgiving them. When you do this, you come into sync with life in time and become able to see and to take advantage of the opportunities for healing and cure that are always arising in and around you. These time debts may be centered in your core, as when they arise through your actions or reactions, or they may be centered outside you, as when they come into you through your parents or community. When you carry time debts that are linked to memories of natural or artificial disasters, you may wish to consult a counselor who can help you to face and resolve them, and thus put them to rest and free you to heal and cure your sevenfold body.

The Web of Life. In sevenfold healing, the web of life is the sum total of all life in the biosphere from the first generative forms of life to the last; it also includes all of the substrates on which life depends. In this view, the human species constitutes a part of the web of life, as does each individual life. This web is interconnected across space and time and is the source and end of all life processes and the tangible and intangible body of all life. The web of life therefore comprises the interconnections through which all life is one.